APPROPRIATE TECHNOLOGY

APPROPRIATE TECHNOLOGY

Articles published in
the *British Medical Journal*

Published by the British Medical Association
Tavistock Square, London WC1H 9JR

© British Medical Journal 1985

All rights reserved. No part of this publication may be reproduced, stored in a retrieval system, or transmitted, in any form or by any means, electronic, mechanical, photocopying, recording and/or otherwise, without the prior written permission of the publishers.

First published 1985

British Library Cataloguing in Publication Data

Appropriate technology
  1 Medical instruments and apparatus—Developing
    countries—Maintenance and repair
  I British Medical Association
  610'.28   R856.5

ISBN-0-7279-0157-5

Printed in England by The Devonshire Press, Barton Road, Torquay.

Preface

"The rich are different from us," said Fitzgerald.
"Nonsense," growled Hemingway. "The rich are the same as us, they just have more money."

The people of the developing world are, by the same token, the same as us, they just have less money. All the more important, then, that they make the best use of every available kwacha or rupee. The fundamentalists of the World Health Organisation urge that resources be directed towards primary health care, to securing a supply of clean water and good sanitation for every village, and these are noble aims. But they ignore the fact that the majority of patients in the wards of a rural district general hospital are likely to be there as a result of trauma, pregnancy, non-waterborne infections, malignancies, and degenerative diseases. They really cannot be left to suffer in the hope that their grandchildren may have a better chance, especially because so many are themselves young adults, the mothers and breadwinners.

The problem is one of apportionment—a problem that taxes the economic experts in this country and is doubly difficult in areas where the national budget may fluctuate wildly, depending on world prices for primary products; where extensive drought may necessitate a quick shift of resources to buy food; and, finally, where there is so little in the way of facts on which to base a programme.

Doctors who work in the Third World are by temperament individualists and inclined to insist that salvation lies in adopting their particular method or organisation even down to their specially designed pharmacopoeias and instrument packs. Yet anyone who has moved from one area to another will find patients treated in different ways, and at very different costs, with equal success. The recent development of simple standard x ray apparatus and laboratory techniques is a recognition of this.

One of the paradoxes of the Third World is that shortages may be so severe that you have to search from one ward to another before you can find a hypodermic needle to give an injection, while the drug store is three quarters filled with useless or grossly out of date and discoloured products. Indeed, it has been estimated that well over half of the expensive apparatus that finds its way to the Third World is lying useless in some dusty corner a few months later, awaiting the arrival of a spare part or knowledgeable technician. Furthermore, vaccines are often rendered ineffective by being left to stew gently in the sun, or given repeatedly to the same child because his previous immunisations were not recorded.

Apart from the material shortages, expatriates who find themselves in a rural district general hospital will suddenly find how much they have taken for granted at home: orderly records; trained pharmacists and the whole chain of people concerned in distribution who ensure that each ward and clinic has its stock of necessary drugs and instruments; laboratories that produce swift and accurate results; physiotherapists, occupational therapists, and a whole army of technicians. The initial despair is later replaced, for those who stick it out, by a realisation that human potential is almost infinite. A lad who left school at the age of 8 may be trained and encouraged to become a first rate radiographer and sound enough radiologist to interpret what he sees and report immediately.

What then are the best systems of organisation, the most efficient techniques, and the "best buys"? Much has already been done to rationalise the provision of drugs, but there is still vast scope for discussion and argument. Should notes be kept centrally or by the patient and in what form so that information is easily retrievable? How many of the

Preface

complex functions undertaken by Western style laboratories are really necessary, or can be reliably exported? Are simple procedures always the most cost effective or would one endoscopist save a hundred or more poor quality radiographs; might ultrasound replace those very x rays, at least in some hospitals, and so on?

One thing is not needed—the Pandora's boxes from which, one eventually finds out, even hope has been omitted. From time to time they arrive, at some far distant railhead, from which they have to be collected and heavy customs duties paid. They then lurk reproachfully in a corner of the drug store until, driven by the hope that something really useful will be discovered in their depths, somebody sets aside a few hours of his or her spare time to unpack them. Several hours later there is a small heap of out of date, second line but potentially still useful antibiotics, a handful of other drugs that might come in useful, and a mound of appetite suppressants, sun creams, vitamin pills, and tranquillisers. "Conscience cartons," they are the modern equivalent of the crumbs cast heedlessly from the rich man's table. We, the Dives of the world, really should do better than that.

ANNE SAVAGE

St Elizabeth's Hospital
Lusikisiki
Transkei
South Africa

Contents

Page

Introduction
Katherine Elliott, MFCM, formerly medical adviser to the Appropriate Health Resources and Technologies Action Group, London 1

Operating theatre and equipment
Peter Bewes, FRCS, consultant surgeon, Birmingham Accident Hospital, Birmingham B15 1NA 3

Immunisation, rehydrations, and transfusion
Katherine Elliott, MFCM, formerly medical adviser to the Appropriate Health Resources and Technologies Action Group, London 6

Diagnostic imaging in small hospitals
P E S Palmer, FRCP, FRCR, professor of radiology, University of California, Davis, CA 95616 9

A plain man's guide to maintenance
Paul Lawrence, BSC, head of technical department, the Joint Mission Hospital Equipment Board, Coulsden, Surrey CR3 2HR 12

Obstetric care
Jill Everett, FRCOG, professor of obstetrics, Faculty of Medicine, University of Papua New Guinea, Boroko, Papua New Guinea 15

Care of the newborn
G J Ebrahim, FRCPED&GLAS, reader in tropical child health, Institute of Child Health, London WC1N 1EH 18

Child health
G J Ebrahim, FRCPED&GLAS, reader in tropical child health, Institute of Child Health, London WC1N 1EN 21

Anaesthetics
F N Prior, FFARCS, consultant anaesthetist, Lewisham Hospital, London SE10 25

Epidemiology and research at low cost
Peter Cox, MD, DTM&H, lecturer in epidemiology, Nuffield Centre for Health Service Studies, Leeds LS2 9PL 29

Priorities for hospital cleaning, disinfection, sterilisation, and control of infection
Rosemary Simpson, MRCPATH, principal microbiologist, Bristol Royal Infirmary 32

Laboratory equipment—where are the tools to do the work?
Monica Cheesbrough, FIMLS, managing director, Tropical Health Technology, Doddington, Cambridgeshire PE15 0TT 35

Equipment for the gastroenterologist
John Nicholls, FRCS, consultant surgeon, Hemel Hemstead General Hospital, Hertfordshire HP2 4AD 40

The cardiologist in the Third World
E G L Wilkins, MRCP, head of department
J I G Strang, MRCP, DTM&H, former principal medical officer, Department of Medicine, Umtata General Hospital, Transkei 43

Contents

The respiratory physician in a Third World district hospital
John Macfarlane, DM, consultant physician, City Hospital, Nottingham 46

Orthopaedic aids at low cost
Ko De Ruÿter and Otto Lelieveld, Department of Physiotherapy, Kasama, Zambia 49

Ophthalmology in developing countries
John Sandford-Smith, FRCS, consultant ophthalmologist, Leicester Royal Infirmary, Leicester LE1 5WW 52

Essential medicines in the Third World
P F D'Arcy, FPS, professor of pharmacy, Queen's University, Belfast 55

Principles of health education
John Hubley, PHD, senior lecturer in health education, Leeds Polytechnic, Leeds 58

Appropriate teaching aids
David Morley, FRCP, professor of tropical child health
Felicity Savage King, MRCP, senior lecturer, Institute of Child Health, London WC1N 1EH 61

Mental health care in the district hospital
H G Egdell, FRCP, MRCPSYCH, consultant psychiatrist, Royal Liverpool Hospital, Liverpool L7 8XP 64

Writing it down
Paul Snell, FRCP, DTM&H, senior registrar in community medicine, Trent Regional Health Authority, Sheffield S10 3TH 68

Index 73

The illustration on the back cover is reproduced by permission of Dr Isabelle de Zoysa.

INTRODUCTION

KATHERINE ELLIOTT

"In our age, the greatest challenge before world medicine is to see that the most useful parts of the knowledge we already have are brought to all those who need it."[1]

Too many millions of people still live brief and disease ridden lives without access to any of the medical benefits already well established. To bridge this gap reliable tools, materials, techniques, and equipment need to be identified, publicised, and made widely available. The chapters in this book aim to identify the technologies needed in the Third World.

No one doubts that medical research will, sooner or later, develop totally new ways to control some of the major tropical diseases but, as their populations increase, the developing countries cannot wait for technological miracles. In many areas more than half of the children die before the age of 5 from a lethal combination of malnutrition and infectious diseases susceptible to simple interventions well within the capacity of the most basic health care services.[2] Until infant and child mortality falls, parents are unlikely to be interested in spacing or limiting their families.

In the long term, better health will depend on socio-economic progress, environmental improvement, and the spread of education. Meanwhile, basic medical care is the immediate need and can also serve as a useful entry point for preventive health care programmes in the community. Even if it were considered desirable (and many of us now question this), there is no way in which the Western pattern of high cost technology and hospital based medical care, supplied by highly trained professionals, could be extended to cover the scattered villages and the crowded urban slum communities where many Third World families live. Their medical care must come through a network of local health workers, who should receive a short, practical training and be given the appropriate equipment for their work. These workers need support in the form of adequate back up facilities at outlying health centres and small district hospitals. This crucial interface is where the genuine appropriateness of many health related technologies will be put to the test.

To be considered appropriate, a technology should meet six criteria. Firstly, it must be effective—that is, it must work and fulfil its purpose in the circumstances in which it needs to be used. Secondly, it must be culturally acceptable and so fit into the hands, minds, and lives of its users without disrupting a social fabric that may already be fragile. (Nevertheless, if new ideas and techniques are introduced they may stimulate local enterprise and promote self sufficiency.) Thirdly, it must be affordable—though this does not imply that an appropriate technology must always be cheap. The trade offs between cost and effectiveness may be worth while, and the choice must be an informed one, made only after full consideration of all the resources that can be made available and the urgency and importance of the need to be met. Fourthly, it must be sustainable locally—that is, the technology should not be overdependent on imported skill for its continuing function, maintenance, and repair. Fifthly, it must be measurable; the impact and performance of any technology needs proper evaluation if it is to be recommended.[3] Finally, it must be politically responsible, for it is unwise to alter an existing balance in a way that might be counterproductive. For example, it might be unwise to encourage minimally trained health workers to take too great an initiative without first making sure that the powerful medical leaders in the area favour this delegation of responsibility and will help the health workers if they run into difficulties.

Techniques and equipment appropriate to the conditions in developing countries must never be stigmatised as second rate just because they may have been superseded in the West. To recall Voltaire, "the best is the enemy of the good."[4] On the other hand, there should be no romanticism about the innate appropriateness of simple technologies. There are already several instances where advanced technologies have provided economical and effective "fixes"—for example, the vaccine safety marker (PATH (Program for Appropriate Technology in Health), Canal Place, 130 Nickerson Street, Seattle, Washington 98104, USA), solar powered refrigeration,[5] and the silver swaddler,[6] which is used to transfer low birthweight babies to a neonatal unit. At the same time, several traditional techniques—for example, acupuncture and an upright position during childbirth—are being evaluated scientifically, so perhaps the transfer of technology ought not to be considered as a one way process.

Some critically annotated lists of best buys among health related apppropriate technologies could provide tremendous support for primary health care movements in all countries and enable those concerned to use their limited resources wisely. In addition, this information may help voluntary agencies and charitable organisations to function

Introduction

more effectively and avoid inappropriate equipment in areas where technical help is urgently needed. These challenges must not be overlooked at a time when so much attention is given to the continuing advance of the frontiers of medical research.

[1] King M. Foreword. In: Elliott K, ed. *The training of auxiliaries in health care (an annotated bibliography)*. London: Intermediate Technology Publications Ltd, 1975.

[2] United Nations Children's Fund. *The state of the world's children*. New York: UNICEF, 1984.

[3] Jequier N. Appropriate technology: the challenge of the second generation. In: Tyrrell DAJ, Henderson W, Elliott K, eds. *More technologies for rural health*. London: Royal Society, 1980.

[4] Voltaire. *Dictionnaire philosophique*. Paris, 1764.

[5] Elliott K. Sun's warmth may keep vaccines cool. *Trop Doct* 1983;**13**: 90–1.

[6] Baum JD, Scopes JW. The silver swaddler: a device for prevention of hypothermia in the newborn. *Lancet* 1968;i:672.

OPERATING THEATRE AND EQUIPMENT

PETER BEWES

I believe that good surgery can be performed in comparatively simple surroundings, which lack the apparently limitless resources of the West, and that it is possible to construct operating theatres where such surgery may be carried out without breaking the bank.

Priorities in allocating funds in surgery

Providing the minimum amount of essential equipment should take precedence over plans for elaborate hospital buildings in areas where resources are limited. A visually splendid hospital without a functioning autoclave or a bronchoscope is clearly a planning disaster. The architectural requirements of a district hospital operating theatre are not necessarily expensive,[1] and local materials may be used for much of the building. Water is so basic to surgery that it must be available readily and this must be borne in mind in the initial decision about where the hospital is to be situated. A hospital that depends on a piped water supply that is not under its own control is vulnerable to the vagaries of the urban water supply, which may totally disrupt surgical services for extended periods. Ideally the operating theatre should have a reasonably large water tank of its own to allow some flexibility when the main hospital tank is depleted for any reason.

Air conditioning may be desirable in hot and humid climates, but it is usually better to ensure that the theatre is kept reasonably cool by attention to architectural detail (adequate roof overhang, proper ventilation etc) rather than by installing an air conditioner that may actually impede the flow of air when—as is so often the case—it breaks down.

Electricity is not essential to the practice of surgery, but it is desirable, for operating the autoclave, the theatre lights, the suction, and the diathermy. There are alternative sources of energy for most of these, however, and diathermy is not essential. If electricity is to be used, a reliable alternative means of generating it must be installed, in case the mains supply fails. This usually implies the installation of a diesel or petrol driven generator.

Sterility

Asepsis is essential to modern surgery, and an autoclave must be regarded as a standard piece of equipment. If there is a source of pressurised steam in the hospital, the autoclave will run off that (fig 1). Where electricity is provided, a semi-automatic electric autoclave such as the Matron made by Surgical Equipment Supplies Ltd is satisfactory. If electricity is not available, an autoclave designed to work on a different type of fuel, such as kerosene, or even charcoal, may be used. Simple boiling does not destroy spores (or even vegetative organisms at high altitudes). It is only in very remote areas that it is necessary to rely solely on chemical means of providing sterility—for example, wringing out the drapes in antiseptic—but these methods may be used successfully.[2]

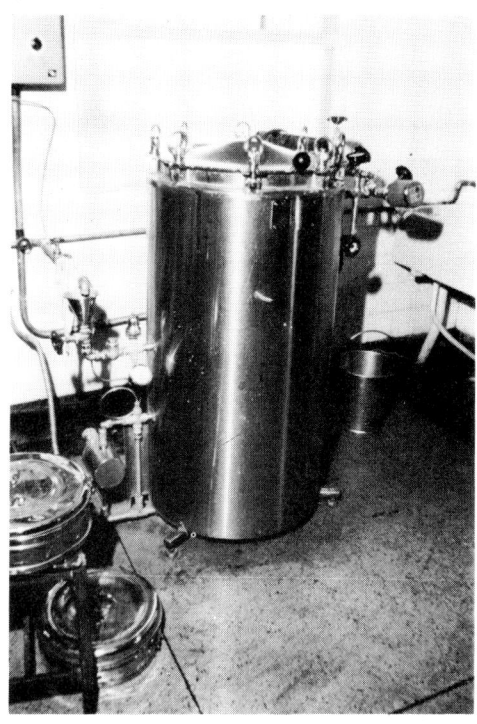

FIG 1—This autoclave is suitable for use where there is a source of steam under pressure. A horizontal autoclave (the electric "Matron" is horizontal) would add some advantages, but at considerable cost, which might not be considered worth the marginal advantage gained.

Lighting

A mistake that is often made is installing complex lights over the operating table, lights that are later found to have bulbs that are almost impossible to trace and reorder when they burn out. While it is possible to operate under a triangle of three fluorescent tubes suspended over the table, a shadowless lamp is better. One of the best patterns (fig 2) has a series of radiating mirrors reflecting light from a single centrally placed bulb. (The Scialytic lamp is a good example.)

Ideally, manufacturers should be encouraged to make a model that uses a standard domestic electric lamp, which is easy to replace. Contrary to popular belief, such a bulb gives a good light,

Operating theatre and equipment

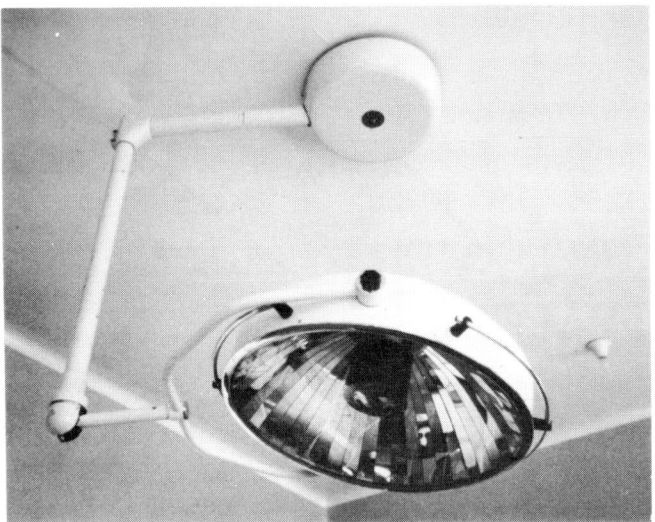

FIG 2—Overhead lamp which is satisfactory for most forms of surgery and may be modified to take household light bulbs.

quite sufficient for operations high under the diaphragm or deep in the pelvis. If the hospital cannot afford a conventional suspension system, the light may be suspended by stout cables from an overhead girder. Alternatively, a floor mounted lamp will have to serve as the main light source.

Operating table

The choice of operating table is critical. If the local repair services cannot maintain the more complex hydraulic types of table, then insist on a simpler pattern. In small hospitals a simple table such as that shown in fig 3 will provide good service for many years, and prove adequate for all the surgery that is likely to be carried out. It also has the advantage of costing only about one hundredth of the cost of the hydraulic table. More expensive tables that still give good value for money include the *Seward Minor* table and the *Thackray Specialist Four*.

Instruments

It is foolish to buy the cheapest equipment; artery forceps are useless if their points do not meet. Kidney dishes should be of stainless steel and not enamel, which does not last so long and soon chips and becomes difficult to clean. Instruments should be simple but good—that is, sharp and well maintained. They should be in use in the teaching hospitals, even though more elaborate equipment may also be present, so that the doctor who proposes to go to work up country has the opportunity to become familiar with them long before he has to use them unsupervised and on his own. For example, excellent skin grafts may be taken with a simple Blair knife (indeed, they have been taken with kitchen knives on occasions), but it is commonplace to hear of hospitals where skin grafting is considered impossible because the residents there have been taught to use only mechanical dermatomes and knives with rollers and disposable blades. I taught myself how to take grafts with a Blair knife, and learnt (from a barber) how to hone and strop it to a keen edge. If there were enough money in all countries to buy Humby knives with their disposable blades, no doubt they would be the best buy; but there isn't, and hence simpler instruments must be purchased.

One or two "general sets" of instruments are sufficient for most operations, and these should be supplemented by special sets for more elaborate procedures. The range of such supplementary sets must be determined by the experience of the surgeon likely to be working in the hospital, but in larger hospitals they might include "specials" such as tracheostomy sets, plastic, gynaecological, urological, thoracic, vascular, and skull instruments. A separate orthopaedic set is also necessary in the larger hospitals. Relatively simple, but good equipment is needed to deal with fractures. Both Jellis and Charnley have argued that non-operative methods may be used in the management of the commoner fractures.[3 4] Jellis goes so far as to say that elaborate apparatus for internal fixation of fractures has no place in an isolated rural hospital. I agree with this view, and believe that in the district hospital no fracture fixation surgery should be undertaken unless the surgeon has adequate orthopaedic experience and has access to good equipment in the form of traction stirrups, Denham pins, and Kirschner wire tensioners (and drills for their easy insertion). Finally, only high quality plaster of paris bandages should be used in the district hospital as it is very difficult to get good results with locally made plaster of paris bandages, even in the hands of the expert, and the expert is not here in the district hospital. We cannot expect a relatively junior doctor to obtain even passable results with a material that his seniors cannot use.

In district general hospitals endoscopes should be available but smaller hospitals will require only facilities for proctoscopy, sigmoidoscopy, culdoscopy, and laryngoscopy. If bronchoscopes, oesophagoscopes, cystoscopes, and gastroscopes are to be ordered, they should share a standard light source with common fittings. It should go without saying that if a certain endoscope is on the list of approved medical stores, then so should be its bulbs, without which it is useless. Where a battery box is necessary for any particular instruments, it should function with the batteries that are likely to be available locally.

Other equipment

I have visited many rural hospitals which boasted a suction machine, but this was rarely in working order. A good argument may thus be made for using a reliable and robust foot operated suction pump based on the car type pump, which will continue to give good service even under adverse circumstances (fig. 4). Diathermy is not essential and should probably be reserved for the more affluent hospitals and those that need to perform thoracic, neurosurgical, and other forms of major surgery.

Prepackaged suture material swaged on to eyeless needles is some 30 000 to 40 000% more expensive than reels of monofilament polyamide (nylon) material bought in bulk. This is suitable for most operations, and spools of suture thread may be mounted on the wall of the room where operation trays are assembled and wrapped. Special suture material should be kept for eye operations and vascular work, and for example, closing the gastric and vesical mucosa.

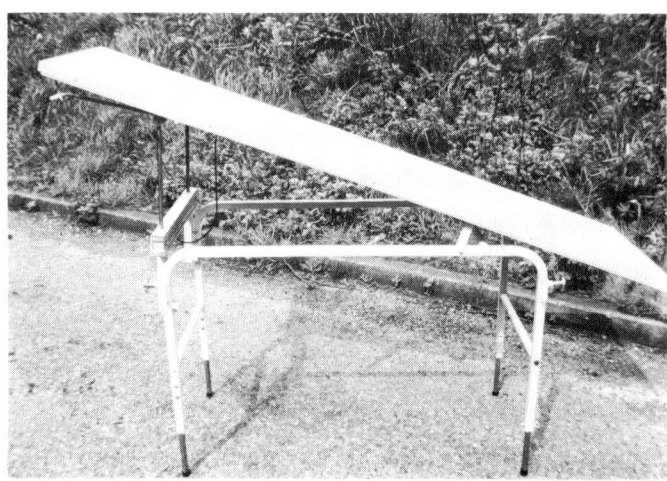

FIG 3—A simple operating table with height and tilt adjustments.

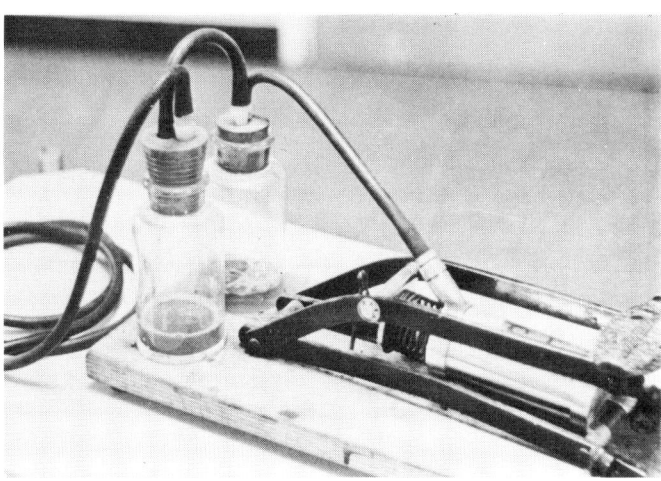

FIG 4—A robust foot operated suction pump modified from a car tyre pump.

An arkansas stone should be available in the theatre suite, so that suture needles, scalpels, and skin graft knives can be reused. A hand sharpened needle will be quite as sharp (and therefore kind to the tissues) as a new eyeless one, and may, on occasions, be even sharper.

Library

Perhaps the most neglected aspect of providing the necessary equipment and facilities for surgery is making provision for a library. A well protected and well kept set of books must be available for the hard pressed doctor who may be called to operate under difficult conditions. Among these I would include Hamilton Bailey's *Emergency Surgery*, A K Henry's *Extensile Exposure*, John Charnley's *Closed Treatment of Common Fractures*, Farquharson's *Operative Surgery*, and F N Prior's *Manual of Anaesthesia*. It is hoped that new texts will be published which are specifically geared to the needs of the isolated general duty doctor working in the operating theatre of a rural hospital.

References

[1] Jorgensen TA. *Proceedings of the Association of Surgeons of East Africa.* 1981;**4**:64-8.
[2] Dick JF. Surgery under adverse conditions. *Lancet* 1966;ii:900-1.
[3] Jellis J. *Proceedings of the Association of Surgeons of East Africa.* 1981; **4**:95-102.
[4] Charnley J. *The closed treatment of common fractures.* 3rd ed. Edinburgh: Churchill Livingstone, 1961.

Recommended reading

Tropical Doctor is a good source and the Christian Medical Fellowship, 157 Waterloo Road, London SE1, sends this free to its members.

KCMC 10th Seminar (Surgery). This may be obtained from the education committee, Kilimanjaro Christian Medical Centre, Private Bag, Moshi, Tanzania, cost £1+postage and packaging.
KCMC 6th Seminar (Anaesthesia), same source as above.

For medical assistants the African Medical Research Foundation, PO Box 30125, Nairobi, Kenya has published a series of manuals on many topics of rural health care. They have a base in London, telephone 01-629 7137.

Reprints of articles for a mission hospital may be obtained from WHO, Avenue Appia, 1211 Geneva 27, Switzerland.

The proceedings of the Association of Surgeons of East Africa, PO Box 8159, Lusaka, Zambia is produced annually and contains useful articles.

IMMUNISATION, REHYDRATION, AND TRANSFUSION

KATHERINE ELLIOTT

To meet the target of Health for All by the Year 2000, set up at Alma-Ata at the joint World Health Organisation (WHO) and United Nations International Children's Emergency Fund (UNICEF) meeting in 1978, all people must have access to effective primary health care. The shape of this health care infrastructure will vary between different countries but is likely to be based on a network of minimally trained community health workers who provide care in the villages and neighbourhoods. As well as training, preferably provided locally, these workers need support from the health centres and small hospitals in their area, and such support must include not only possibilities for supervision and referral but also a whole range of really appropriate health related technologies—the tools needed to carry out the tasks.

This back up for community health workers is essential, and the conventional health services must act as staging posts where essential materials may be prepared or received and safely stored on arrival from central depots, ready for use or for further distribution to the periphery. In 1983 UNICEF, in response to its report on the state of the world's children, declared that it intended to concentrate on four major aspects of child health: breast feeding, growth monitoring, immunisation, and oral rehydration. It should not, however, be forgotten that, when growth monitoring indicates the need, nutritional support ought to be made available as part of primary health care. Similarly, oral rehydration programmes, which undoubtedly prevent many unnecessary deaths from dehydration, remain only a panacea unless they can be combined with improvements in water supplies, sanitation, and community education in environmental hygiene. Nevertheless, UNICEF and WHO are working closely together to expand and extend oral rehydration and immunisation programmes to cover even the most remote areas. Both types of programmes have technological implications for the health centre and small district hospital.

Immunisation

Immunisation services should be provided as an integral part of a primary health care system, and immunisation coverage is both a simple and an important indicator of that system's success. The technologies concerned in providing such a service consist of the provision of effective vaccines, when and where they are to be used, combined with the knowledge of how vaccines may be safely stored and transported and used. The most successful immunisation programmes are those that are carried out with maximum community participation in planning, implementation, and evaluation.[1] Those concerned with providing immunisation services must reckon with the realities of available vaccines as well as the local skills to implement the programme.

The success of the smallpox eradication programme was helped by the development of a heat stable, freeze dried vaccine, the use of the bifurcated needle which could be sterilised easily and used again in multiple pressure vaccination, and the surveillance by WHO reference laboratories of the quality of vaccine from different sources. Cleaning the skin before vaccination was found to be unnecessary, and so the vaccinator's total equipment could be carried in one pocket—two small plastic tubes for needles plus vaccine and a diluent.

Measles immunisation of young infants in high risk areas may soon to be possible using a new aerosol vaccine, which can be sprayed into the upper respiratory tract. Babies inherit some protection against measles from their mothers but, where measles is a particularly common and serious infection, this protection may not last until the normal age (9–10 months) for measles immunisation is reached. The new vaccine could be a valuable step forward in child survival in developing countries and results from its field trials are being eagerly awaited.[2] Work is also being done to produce less fragile vaccines for use against other major communicable diseases—for example, a freeze dried diphtheria/pertussis/tetanus (DPT) vaccine. New immunisation schedules are being developed to reduce the number of visits necessary by combining inactivated and live vaccines for simultaneous administration, or by decreasing the need for additional inoculations by conferring more effective protection initially. Meanwhile, until advanced laboratory technology has managed to produce a one shot vaccine that will remain potent in any health worker's pocket, problems of transport and storage of vaccine remain a matter of concern. The vaccines that are currently used need to be kept at appropriate temperatures around freezing point at all stages in their journey from the point of manufacture right up to their point of entry into the person who is being immunised.

Refrigeration

In the health centre or small district hospital vaccine safety is likely to depend on domestic refrigerators powered by electricity, gas, or kerosene. Electricity in rural areas is often unreliable or non-existent. Supplies of bottled gas and kerosene depend on transport facilities and are affected by road conditions and pilferage. Kerosene refrigerators require careful maintenance to keep them functioning efficiently. There is also the temptation to use some of the limited refrigeration space for perishable foods and cold drinks (an understandable weakness in places where ambient temperatures are uncomfortably high and there is no other method of cooling things), but a refrigerator frequently opened is not a safe place for vaccines. These must be placed within their own special refrigerator because DPT, tetanus toxoid, and BCG vaccines need to be stored at 4-8°C

Immunisation, rehydration, and transfusion

and never frozen, whereas measles and polio vaccines should be kept below 0°C in the freezing compartment.

The refrigerator must also provide the ice required for the transport of vaccines to outlying clinics and health posts. Vaccines should be carried in cold boxes and in vacuum flask type carriers. In these containers vaccines must be kept cool by packing them with commercial ice packs or bags of ice cubes. Good supplies of ice are, therefore, essential for efficient immunisation. A properly made, well insulated cold box containing sufficient quantities of ice will keep vaccines safe for up to four days, provided that it is kept in the shade and not opened too often. Refrigeration plays a crucial part in immunisation and is not susceptible to improvisation.

Recent advances

Technology may contribute to success of immunisation in various ways: firstly, by improving refrigerator design—for example, top rather than front opening entails less cold loss, and simple improvements to the gas or kerosene burner unit may make maintenance easier—and, secondly, by developing alternative power sources for refrigeration such as solar power, which has the potential for higher performance, lower running costs, improved reliability, and a longer working life than conventionally powered refrigerators. A solar powered refrigerator/freezer for storing vaccines is being tested by the Lewis Research Centre of the National Aeronautics and Space Administration of the United States of America in collaboration with the WHO in six countries, starting in India.[3] Research is also being carried out at other centres on a whole range of different approaches to solar powered refrigeration (fig 1). Its success may make a major contribution to the refrigeration requirements of small hospitals and health centres, as it makes use of a free and freely available source of power.

The success of any immunisation programme depends on the integrity of the "cold chain" between central store, district hospital, health centre, and the community. Technology has made effective monitoring of the cold chain's integrity possible by producing a vaccine safety marker. This is a heat sensitive indicator to monitor the time and temperature history of individual phials of vaccine. The indicator consists of a small circular paper tab, with adhesive backing and protective coating, which is applied to individual vaccine phials on the flip off part of the cap, either at the central store or at the site of manufacture

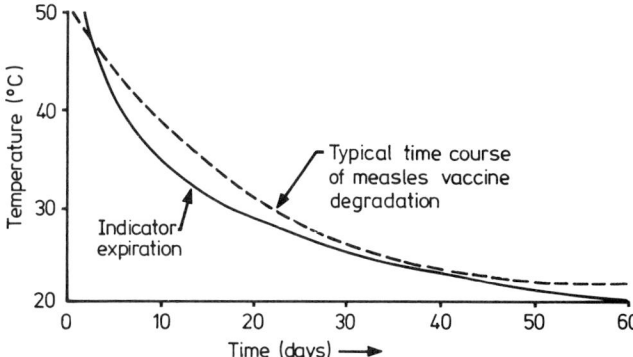

FIG 2—Freeze dried measles vaccine may be stored safely for 1-2 years at 2-8°C, but when exposed to 37°C the potency falls below acceptable levels within 1-2 weeks. The degradation of the indicator parallels the rate of decline of the vaccine, and it changes colour after exposure to a critical accumulation of time and temperature.

of the vaccine. Developed by PATH (Program for Appropriate Technology in Health),[4] the marker is based on a polymer that changes colour from red to black when exposed to a critical accumulation of time and temperature. The rate of colour change parallels, but on the conservative side, the rate of decline towards minimum potency of the vaccine, rapidly changing from an initial safe red to danger black when the vaccine should not be used. Darkening of the red suggests that the vaccine should be used without delay. At present the marker is adjusted for measles vaccine (which is notoriously fragile, see fig 2), and costs less than 10% of a 10 dose phial of measles vaccine. The marker is being tested in the field, and work is under way to adapt the basic principle for use with other vaccines, starting with polio. The London School of Hygiene and Tropical Medicine, the International Development Research Centre in Canada, the Edna McConnell Clark Foundation, and the WHO have all collaborated with PATH to develop the vaccine safety marker. It is an excellent example of the imaginative application of modern technology to solve a problem that usually arises in remote circumstances where the cold chain is most likely to be broken.

Fluid replacement

Of the four major interventions that UNICEF is promoting, oral rehydration has the greatest immediate potential for saving life.[5] [6] Diarrhoea kills at least five million children every year in the Third World and contributes to the ill health and malnutrition of countless others who survive. In diarrhoea, dehydration is the lethal factor, and since the early 1970s it has been known that the fluids and electrolytes that are lost may usually be replaced satisfactorily by mouth instead of intravenously. This therapeutic advance is based on the discovery that glucose aids intestinal absorption of sodium, thus hastening the restoration of fluid balance. The formula recommended by WHO for oral rehydration salts solution is as follows: sodium chloride 3·5 g, trisodium citrate dihydrate 2·9 g (or sodium bicarbonate 2·5 g), potassium chloride 1·5 g, glucose 20 g. These quantities are mixed with one litre of (preferably) safe water.

Another change, and another possible improvement in the ORS formula, may come from recent rehydration studies where rice powder has been substituted for the glucose or sucrose. The preliminary results are encouraging.[7] Other alternative carbohydrate sources, such as wheat, maize, millet, sorghum, and potato, are being investigated. Work is also taking place to develop enriched oral rehydration solutions,[8] to which amino acids like glycine, for example, or peptides have been added to promote earlier and more effective refeeding in diarrhoea.

Sachets or packets of oral rehydration salts (ORS) may be kept at the district hospital and distributed to the smaller hospitals

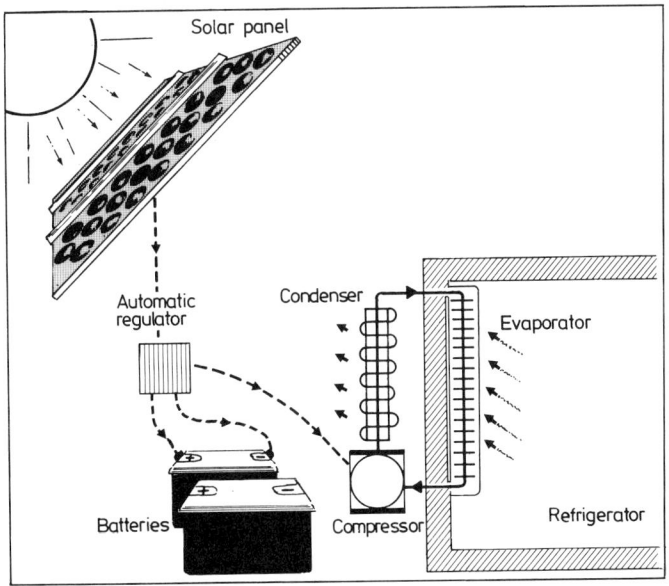

FIG 1—Schematic representation of how a solar powered refrigerator works.

Immunisation, rehydration, and transfusion

and health centres. The full formula, if it contains sodium bicarbonate, needs to be packaged in foil or freshly made up from the separate ingredients. The replacement of bicarbonate by citrate in the ORS formula is the result of laboratory studies by the WHO diarrhoeal diseases programme, followed by extensive clinical trials.[9] The ORS-citrate formula is possibly even more effective and it is more stable, thus permitting the use of less expensive packaging material and giving ORS packets a longer shelf life. In many areas supply systems for the distribution of ORS packets are subject to frequent breakdowns and it is essential to teach families how to make up simple sugar and salt solutions for use in home-based treatment. Mothers also need to be taught about the importance of breast feeding and the early restarting of other feeding after any episode of diarrhoea.

In areas where oral rehydration programmes have been established successfully the need for parenteral fluids is reduced, but intravenous fluids are still needed for children with gross hypovolaemia. Intraperitoneal fluids are also sometimes given in certain circumstances. Such fluids must, therefore, be readily available. Apart from their use in cases of severe dehydration they are also needed to treat patients with trauma, obstetric haemorrhage, the need for emergency surgery, and so on. Saline based fluids are perhaps most efficiently produced at a central health facility, but they are heavy, bulky, and expensive to transport and have a limited shelf life of three to six months. They may be made at small hospitals provided that scrupulous care is taken to avoid contamination. Ingredients must be pure and measured out accurately. An abundant supply of distilled water is essential, and the design of efficient stills for this purpose is important.

Appropriate technology

Stills are probably best made of glass and heated by any convenient source of energy—electricity, gas, or kerosene (the development of solar powered stills would be an advantage in many areas). The risk of contamination with pyrogens is reduced if the distilled water is filtered through an easily cleaned sintered glass filter. Plastic rather than rubber connections are recommended, but rubber bung seals for the bottles remain essential. These are still available from some manufacturers and are almost infinitely reusable, as are the glass bottles. Disposable plastic giving sets should be used, not rubber tubing. Efficient autoclaves are another essential, and here again, as with stills, appropriate technological interests should be enlisted with regard to design, power sources, and easy maintenance. Any risk of contamination should be slight provided that sufficient care is taken at all stages, including the cleaning of all apparatus. Staff who take on this responsibility at the periphery must receive proper training, which may best be undertaken centrally.

As with all other forms of training for workers at the periphery, the central staff concerned should have had realistic experience of working there themselves.

Plasma and blood

Plasma cannot be prepared locally, but freeze dried plasma has a long life if kept in a refrigerator. It may be reconstituted as required using freshly prepared and filtered distilled water. Blood supplies frequently come from a central blood bank and can be stored safely in a refrigerator for up to 21 days at a temperature that does not exceed 4°C. Blood grouping and cross matching must also be available, and therefore blood may be collected locally at health centres or small hospitals, using containers as prepared for other intravenous fluids. Again, it is recommended that prepacked plastic disposable taking and giving sets should be used. As it is already recognised that plastic disposable syringes are often resterilised for multiple use, however, research ought to be done into all so called disposable equipment to establish how and how often it may safely be reused.

Sterilisation of some types of equipment may be improvised—for example, syringes and needles, some instruments, and ligatures may be simply boiled in any container over any source of heat—although autoclaving is essential for many purposes. PATH has developed a sterilisation safety marker, which is being tested in the field. It consists of a coloured plastic disc protected by a metal ring. The colour changes when the disc has been kept at a temperature of 100°C for not less than 20 minutes. The disc is reusable and cheap and should be a useful way to check the adequacy of sterilisation by boiling, as for instance in home deliveries or in field conditions for immunisation.

Adequate storage facilities in hospitals and health centres are essential, and there are several simple ways in which they may be readily improved. A useful handbook has been published by AHRTAG called *How to look after a health centre store*.[10] This makes a good companion volume to their other publications, *How to look after a refrigerator* and *How to make a cold box*. Undoubtedly efficient refrigeration is crucial for the proper functioning of any medical centre, not only for the storage and transport of vaccine but also for the safe storage of serum; antitoxin; reconstituted antibiotics for injection; drugs such as some forms of insulin; and, finally, plasma and blood.

To look at immunisation, rehydration, and transfusion as peripheral procedures, clearly there is great scope for modification of existing methods and the imaginative application of appropriate technologies.

References

[1] Training manuals available from the expanded programme for immunisation (EPI), WHO, 1211 Geneva 27, Switzerland.
[2] Sabin AB, Arechiga AF, de Castro JF, *et al*. Successful immunisation of children with and without maternal antibody by aerosolized measles vaccine. *JAMA* 1983;**249**:2651-62.
[3] Elliott K. Sun's warmth may keep vaccines cool. *Trop Doct* 1983;**13**:90-1.
[4] PATH (Program for Appropriate Technology in Health), Canal Place, 130 Nickerson Street, Seattle, Washington 98109, USA.
[5] Anonymous. Oral rehydration: the time has come. *Lancet* 1983;ii:259.
[6] Elliott K, Cutting WAM, eds. *Diarrhoea Dialogue* (Quarterly newsletter, free to developing countries from 85 Marylebone High Street, London W1M 3DE).
[7] Patra FC, Mahalamabis D, Jalan KN, Sen A, Banerjee P. Is oral rice electrolyte solution superior to glucose electrolyte solution in infantile diarrhoea? *Arch Dis Child* 1982;**57**:910-2.
[8] Patra FC, Mahalamabis D, Jalan KN, Sen A, Banerjee P. In search of a super solution: controlled trial of glycine-glucose oral rehydration solution in infantile diarrhoea. *Paediatrica Scandinavia* 1984;**73**:18-21.
[9] Guidelines for the Production of Oral Rehydration Salts (document WHO/CDD/SER/80.3), 1984 revised version available from the Director, Diarrhoea Diseases Control Programme, WHO, 1211 Geneva 27, Switzerland.
[10] AHRTAG (Appropriate Health Resources and Technologies Action Group). *How to look after a refrigerator. How to look after a health centre store. How to make a cold box*. From AHRTAG, 85 Marylebone High Street, London W1M 3DE.

DIAGNOSTIC IMAGING IN SMALL HOSPITALS

P E S PALMER

How do you choose equipment for imaging from the bewildering and tempting array of alternatives, particularly when your budget is limited? The rules for shopping for images are the same as those for shopping in a supermarket: have a clear idea of what you need, and remember that cheapness may be a false economy.

Imaging for the non-radiologist in a small hospital means diagnostic x ray equipment or ultrasound or both. Ultrasound is extremely useful for looking at structures within the abdomen, for obstetrics, and for visualising the liver and abdominal and pelvic masses. It may also provide information about the kidney, pancreas, and gall bladder. There are no radiation hazards (so far as is known) and imaging is easy, although recording the image is more difficult and expensive. The main disadvantage is that ultrasound is time consuming for the physician as the work cannot be delegated.

X ray equipment has much wider application: in all cases of trauma, in many infections, especially those in the chest, in intestinal obstruction, in the investigation of genitourinary and gall bladder disease, and in obstetric practice. Apart from its wider usefulness, the work may be delegated to paramedical staff and there is a permanent record. The disadvantages are costs (US $25 000 upwards compared with $10 000 upwards for ultrasound) and the hazard of radiation, which may be controlled easily with proper precautions.

If you have the alternative, buy x ray equipment only. The use for ultrasound in a small hospital is so limited that money should be saved to purchase an x ray set.

X ray equipment

Any x ray installation requires an x ray set (generator, control, tube, and support for the patient); a darkroom with processing tanks, chemicals, cassettes, and films; and essential extras such as lead aprons, lead gloves, x ray viewing boxes, and film envelopes.

Provided properly designed equipment, such as the World Health Organisation Basic Radiological System (fig 1) is chosen, there is no need to have elaborate rooms with thick walls and lead doors. Local materials may be used; a firm and fairly flat floor is essential, and the ceiling height must be not less than 2·5 m. The room must be weatherproof, well ventilated, and at least 18 m². There must be easy access for beds and trolleys. The darkroom must be nearby, about 5 m², preferably with running water. A small storeroom or office of about 8 m² is helpful.

The World Health Organisation recommends a fixed generator (as opposed to a mobile, "portable," or "ward" unit) with not less than 11 kW output. Specify this power, not less, because this is the minimum that will provide good quality chest x ray films as well as good radiographs of adult lumbar spines, the abdomen, and the fetus.

A mobile unit is unsatisfactory because it increases the radiation risks to staff and patients, operator training is more difficult, and the results are more variable. The only disadvantage of a fixed unit is for patients who are immobilised: they must be brought to the x ray department in their beds.

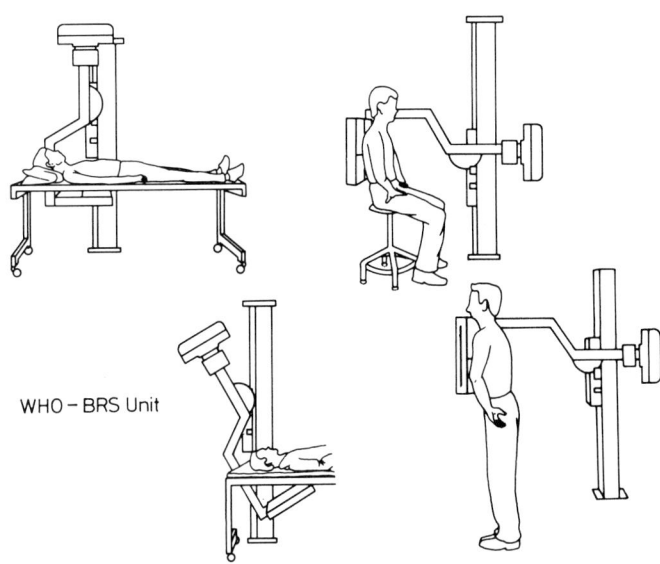

FIG 1—The design of the WHO Basic Radiological System permits 100 standard projections with simplicity yet accuracy. 11 kW is the minimum power requirement.

WHAT ELECTRICAL POWER IS REQUIRED?

If there is a small local electrical generator, an unreliable power supply, or a long cable from the nearest transformer choose a battery operated unit, but still of 11 kW. These may be recharged continuously from any 5 amp wall outlet (110 V or 220 V), and they go on working throughout the day even if the hospital generator operates only at night or if the main electrical supply is turned off at any time. Condenser discharge units are not satisfactory. They can produce satisfactory chest x ray films, but the spine or abdomen and pregnant women may have an x ray examination only at the expense of increased radiation and decreased quality. They need a constant electrical supply. They are an unacceptable alternative to an 11 kW fixed unit.

Diagnostic imaging in small hospitals

WHO CAN OPERATE AN X RAY UNIT?

If the World Health Organisation Basic Radiological System is chosen anyone with a primary school education and preferably some previous hospital experience—for example, an orderly, nurse aid, assistant nurse, or lab technician—may learn to use it in a few weeks. WHO produces a simple step by step manual that covers all the necessary *x* ray examinations for a busy hospital (fig 2). Special techniques are shown for children. There is a section on patient care and radiation protection for staff and patients. The operator should first be taught at a large hospital by trained radiographers; this usually takes from two weeks to three months depending on the individual. With the basic radiological system such an operator may examine from three to 20 patients per day—with the help of a darkroom technician even more.

THE DARKROOM

A small truly "dark" room with running water and electric light is essential. A design for the film processing tank is shown in fig 3. The outside tank is best made out of high quality stainless steel that resists chemicals (ordinary stainless steel will survive about three months). Alternatively, the tank may be made of cement and preferably tiled. It is helpful to have hot water available if the ambient temperature drops below 20°C. Provided the appropriate chemicals are used, there is no need to have any method of cooling the processing tanks. The inner tanks, for developer and fixer, usually have about a 25 l capacity and should be of the appropriate quality of stainless steel. Plastic insert tanks are available, but they warp and have a relatively short life. Smaller self contained processing units are available with a 15 l capacity for developer and fixer, but these are suitable only for three to five patients per day.

X RAY FILMS AND CASSETTES

There are many different makes of *x* ray film, all of different speeds and quality. Usually the faster the film the poorer the quality of image. *X* ray films go between fluorescent screens inside cassettes, which must be lightproof and made of plastic or steel. Buy the best you can afford. Good cassettes will last 10 years in a small hospital and screens about five years. The fluorescent screens also come in many varieties of speed and quality. With an 11 kW generator choose a medium or standard speed rather than an ultra fast one. WHO recommends two sizes at least, 35 × 43 cm and 24 × 30 cm. Not more than two additional film sizes may be chosen, but make sure that these cassette sizes match the collimator (the beam limiting system)

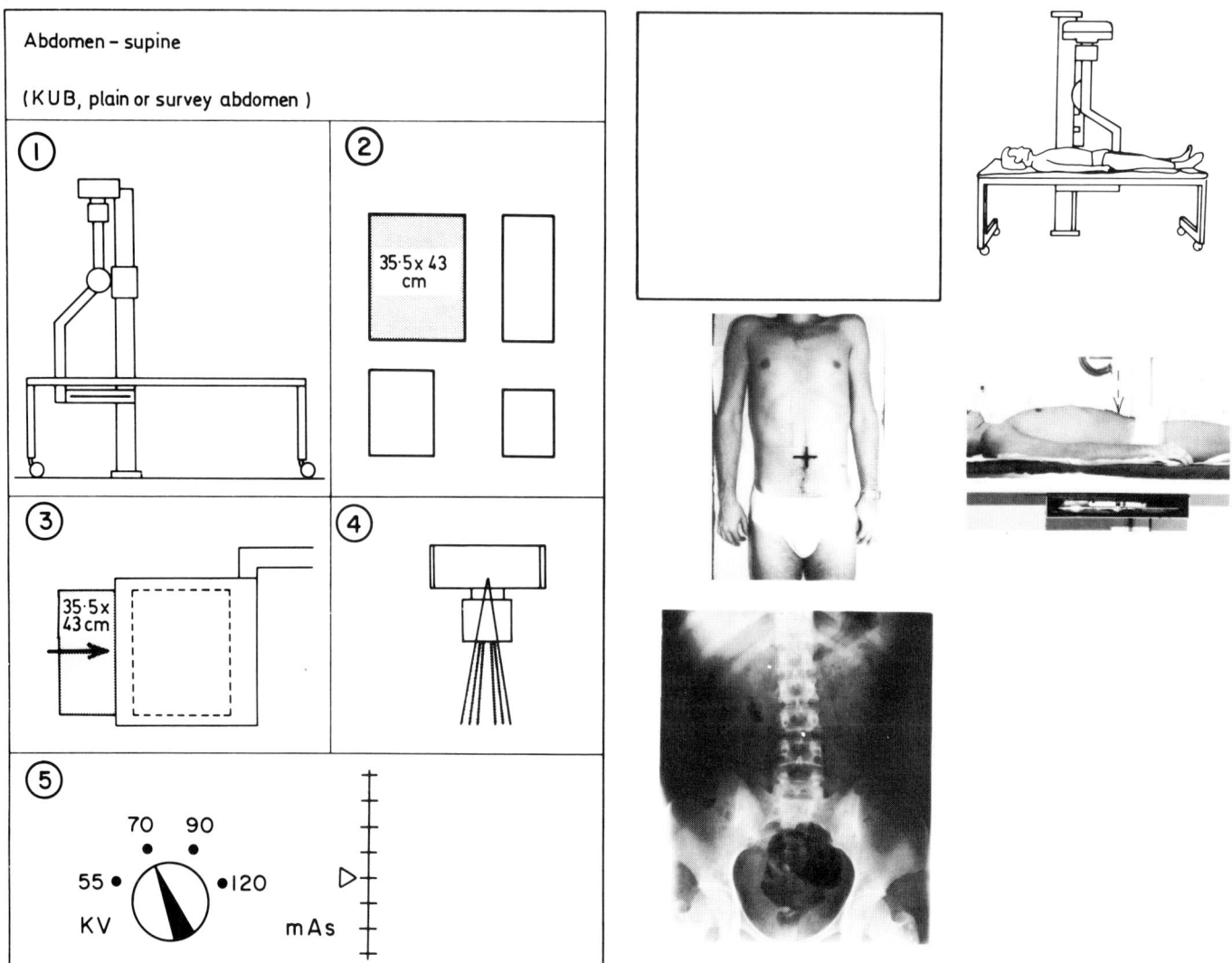

FIG 2—Left and right pages from the WHO *Manual of Radiographic Technique*. Space is available at the top of each page to write in additional instructions or reminders in the local language.

Diagnostic imaging in small hospitals

of the x ray unit. One of the major disadvantages of a mobile unit is an inaccurate beam; this decreases quality and increases radiation hazards.

INSTALLATION AND COSTS

The manufacturer will install the machine, then an experienced radiographer must come to set the exposure charts or controls, using the film, screens, and processing chemicals

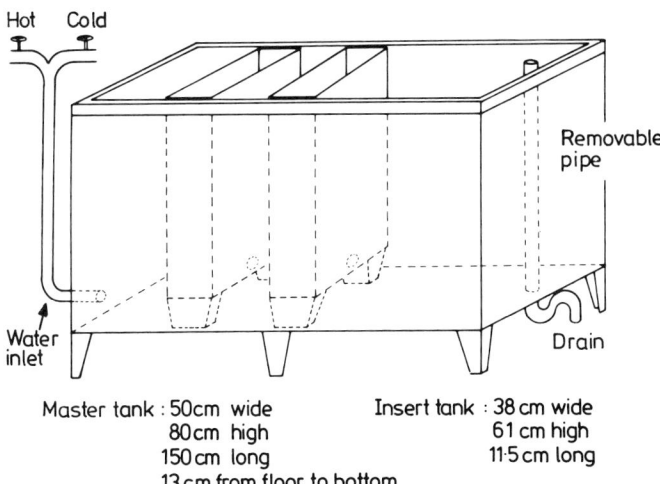

FIG 3—The WHO Basic Radiological System pattern for a simple x ray processing tank. As the number of patients increase additional chemical tanks can be added to this unit.

Master tank: 50 cm wide, 80 cm high, 150 cm long, 13 cm from floor to bottom
Insert tank: 38 cm wide, 61 cm high, 11·5 cm long

in your hospital. These cannot be preset in the factory. The exposures will then remain satisfactory until the type of film or screen is changed, when the exposure charts or controls must be recalibrated. At current costs, a satisfactory complete x ray installation complying with WHO's specifications, and providing the darkroom equipment and all the accessories, costs about $25 000. (Obviously these prices vary with different manufacturers and countries.) Do not, however, choose only by price: look carefully at the back up that is available. Is the manufacturer selling you equipment or does it come from "agents"? In general, beware of agents; experience suggests that the ability to sell x ray machines does not necessarily include a scholarly knowledge of x ray equipment. Similarly, choose x ray films that are similar to those in the larger hospitals in your country rather than an apparently cheaper supply from the local store.

Ultrasound

As with x ray sets, ultrasound comes in small, large, simple complex, cheap ($10 000), and expensive ($80 000 or more) varieties.

An entirely satisfactory ultrasound imaging unit, the size of a small suitcase and just as portable, is available for about $10 000; this will produce a black and white image on a small screen and needs a 5 amp AC source at 110 V or 220 V. It has simple control knobs. Four weeks spent in a busy ultrasound department will allow an inexperienced doctor to recognise most of the important obstetric problems; any large tumour, cyst, or abscess in the liver or spleen or kidney; a swollen pancreas, a pancreatic pseudocyst; an ovarian, dermoid, or other pelvic tumour; and a sizable pelvic or peritoneal abscess or mass. With practice, the gall bladder, calculi, and obstructed bile ducts may be recognised and aortic aneurysms defined. Any diagnostic skills beyond these require much more training. It is important to remember that a physician will have to carry out each and every patient examination, and there is no place for the part time or occasional ultrasound technician.

LIMITATIONS AND COSTS

A permanent record is needed but recording the image from a small screen can be a problem. A camera using a self developing (Polaroid or similar) film is available. These work well, but the film is not cheap and the camera is expensive. Even more expensive cameras use standard x ray film. Measuring the image on the screen directly with callipers is a compromise that is not accurate and not reproducible. Recently (1985) the small photocopier has become available for this purpose, which produces a satisfactory image on cheap paper: currently (1985) this costs about $300 and the paper is under $20.00 for about 1000 images. This is a good solution to the need to have a permanent image.

The design and production of ultrasound equipment are changing rapidly: any description now will be out of date before this article is printed. The description above provides a basis from which your requirements may be specified. WHO (1985) can supply detailed specifications for an ultrasound unit for small hospitals, particularly in developing countries, which were drawn up by an international scientific group which met at the end of 1984. Despite the persuasive stories of those selling you these equipment, stick with the WHO specifications, neither more nor less, and you will have an entirely satisfactory ultrasound unit which will do all or even more than you can possibly need. However, choose the supplier and the manufacturer with the same care as you would an x ray set.

If you have limited money use a great deal of caution—a non-functioning $10 000 ultrasound unit is a frustrating item and it is not even decorative. The WHO scientific group emphasised that the first need of a small hospital is an x ray unit and that ultrasound is an additional luxury.

Although I hope that this article reflects the views of the whole WHO expert group (Radiology in the Developing Countries), all of whom have many years of practical experience with the difficulties of imaging in small hospitals, I must take personal responsibility for the opinions expressed. Dr N Racoveanu, chief of radiation medicine, World Health Organisation, Geneva, and his office will respond to requests for advice or specifications or refer the inquiry to one of the WHO advisers.

Recommended reading

Radiology and primary care. 1978. (Pan American Health Organisation Scientific Publication No 357.) Pan American Health Organisation, NW Washington, DC 20037.

Radiology and basic care hospitals and clinics. In: Kleczkowski BM, Pibouleau R, eds. *Approaches to planning and design of health care facilities in developing areas.* Vol 3. Geneva: WHO, 1979:83-124. (WHO Offset Publication No 45.)

The WHO-BRS manual of radiographic technique. Geneva: WHO, 1984.

The WHO-BRS manual of darkroom technique. Geneva: WHO, 1984.

The WHO-BRS diagnostic manual for primary care physicians. Geneva: WHO, 1984.

Palmer PES, ed. Radiology in the developing world. Diagnostic imaging. *Journal of the Netherlands Society of Radiodiagnosis* 1982;51:117-200.

Cockshott P, Middlemiss H. *Clinical radiology in the tropics.* Edinburgh: Churchill Livingstone, 1979.

Reeder M, Palmer PES. *The radiology of tropical diseases.* Baltimore: Williams and Wilkins, 1981.

A PLAIN MAN'S GUIDE TO MAINTENANCE

PAUL LAWRANCE

Hospitals house a variety of equipment, and it would be inappropriate in this article to give detailed maintenance schedules for any particular items. Instead, I intend to try to present a practical approach from my own experience of maintaining and repairing equipment in developing countries. As a general principle it is wise to adhere to the manufacturer's recommendations whenever possible, but this is a counsel of perfection that is seldom easy to follow because of lack of information, spare parts, or, simply, time.

New equipment: a cautionary approach

A lot of time and energy may be saved by choosing suitable equipment at the outset. Factors to be borne in mind should include the degree of local skill (do the people who are to use and maintain the machine understand its basic working principles ?), the harshness of the local environment (humidity, temperature stability, and conditions of electrical supply), and whether spare parts are readily available. Irrespective of long term availability, it is a good idea to purchase a stock of spare parts when you buy the equipment (manufacturers will normally provide a list of suggested spares on request), and ensure that manuals and clear diagrams for identifying spare parts are supplied with the equipment. I have heard of many instances where this has not been the case, and the delay in obtaining information may lead to continuous correspondence culminating in a frustrating reply such as "the equipment is now obsolete."

It is not always wise to choose the most modern equipment, for its impressive veneer may have been achieved in exchange for simplicity, ruggedness, and reliability. Purchasing several machines of the same type simplifies maintenance as spares for only one model are necessary and in a crisis parts from one may be used in another; also, maintenance staff need only to understand how one model works.

When a new piece of equipment is bought the manuals should be read through and thoroughly understood before it is installed. We have a poster in our office which admirably illustrates this point (fig 1). A log should be kept for each piece of equipment; this will help in recognising repetitive faults and simplify your judgment as to when a component should be left alone, cleaned, or replaced. The log should include the date of purchase, the times when the equipment is in use, the initials of the maintenance staff, and details of all faults reported and any maintenance work carried out. Ideally, routine maintenance is undertaken, and where several machines are used a wall chart similar to the one shown in figure 2 may prove useful.

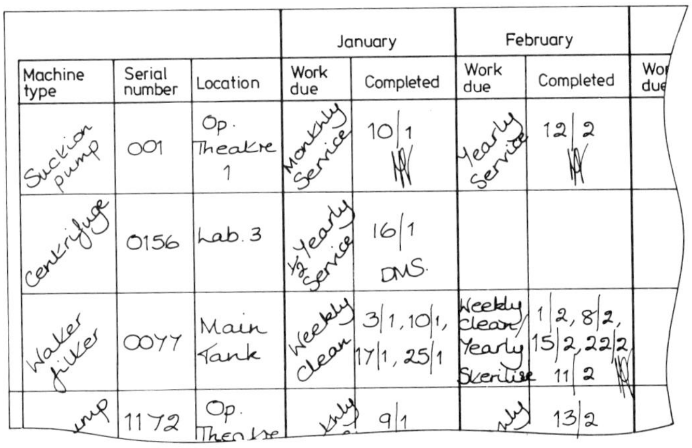

			January		February		
Machine type	Serial number	Location	Work due	Completed	Work due	Completed	Wo[rk] due
Suction pump	001	Op. Theatre 1	Monthly Service	10/1	Yearly Service	12/2	
Centrifuge	0156	Lab. 3	½ Yearly Service	16/1 DMS.			
Water filter	0077	Main Tank	Weekly clean	3/1, 10/1, 17/1, 25/1	Weekly clean/ Yearly Sterilise	1/2, 8/2, 15/2, 22/2, 11/2	
...mp	1172	Op. Theatre	...thly	9/1	...ly	13/2	

FIG 2—Wall chart showing maintenance schedules.

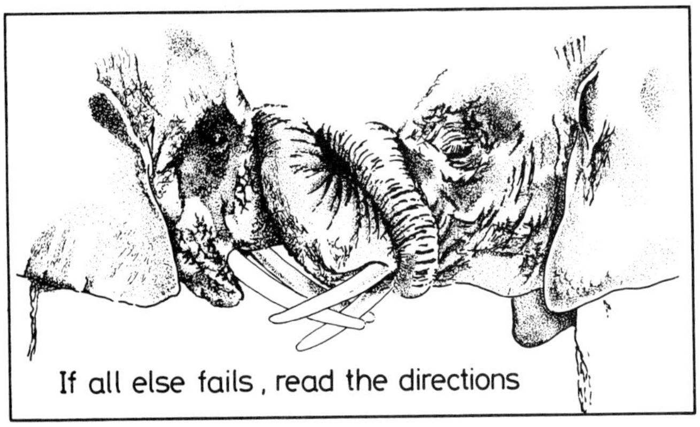

FIG 1—Aide-mémoire for dealing with new items of equipment.

Personnel for repair and maintenance

If the equipment for the hospital has been chosen wisely so that it is simple to understand, the technical knowledge required to repair it will be reduced. Many of the faults I have encountered in the Third World have been extremely simple to diagnose and repair. Most faults require simply an adjustment or an item cleaned out or lubricated, while others can be repaired with a minimum of tools and spare parts. Perhaps it is worth considering asking your laboratory technician to take a look at some of the faults on equipment other than those in his domain. The main requirements are for a systematic approach and a little self confidence. I would say as a cautionary note that it would be foolhardy for an untrained person to tackle an *x* ray machine or equipment of similar complexity, other than to check fuses and electrical connections.

Much of the simple preventative maintenance can be completed by untrained staff. All that is required is a reliable character who you know will wash the filter every month, top up the lubricant weekly, etc. For this routine work an inquiring mind can be a hindrance rather than a help as the work involves following a set procedure. Thus, the people required for maintenance are not necessarily the same as those required for repair. They do not have to understand the working of the machine, but in this case they must not tamper with the equipment and should just follow the set procedure precisely.

Importance of preventive maintenance

Preventive maintenance is preferable to waiting until the components require emergency repair or replacement—both for convenience and for patient safety. Thus, although it may appear unnecessary to take a working pump out of operation for maintenance, a day or two of lost use may prevent total failure of the pump in a few months' time. When you carry out preventive maintenance, apart from repairing faulty components you should replace components that are suspect or likely to fail, owing to their age, before the next service. As a rough guide, if you plot the likelihood of a component's failure against time a bath shaped graph results (fig 3). The time at which a component is replaced should be before the upturn of the graph; this time will clearly depend on the part itself, its environment, and how much the equipment is used. Replacing components before they fail may prevent other, more expensive, items failing.

Ample time is needed for preventive maintenance and subsequent testing. Trying to repair a piece of equipment with a doctor breathing down your neck waiting to use it is sometimes inevitable but is likely to be detrimental to both the maintenance staff and the next patient. Ideally, a mutually convenient time should be set aside by both the user and the maintainer so that they may look at the equipment together. This provides a perfect opportunity of gaining insight into how the equipment is performing. The operators may have noticed a slightly different noise from usual or a symptom of a fault that, while not important enough to warrant immediate attention, may be rectified easily. In a complete breakdown, a history of problems may help in diagnosis (a familiar concept for doctors and maintenance staff alike).

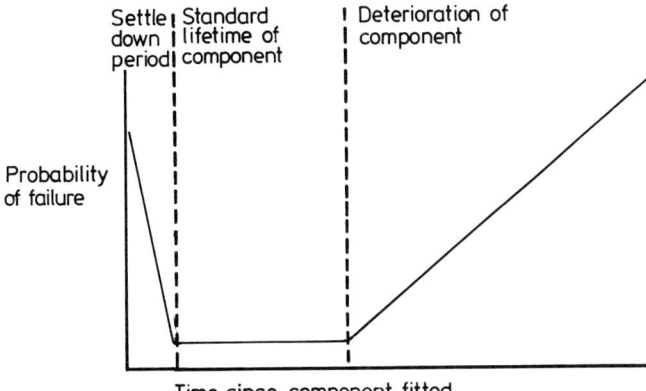

FIG 3—Rough guide to predict the life span of an individual component of a machine.

How to go about it

Before embarking on any maintenance work avoid the risk of infection; always assume that the equipment is unsterile and use protective gloves and a mask if these are available. For similar reasons of self preservation, check that the equipment is electrically and mechanically safe to work on. For example, with electrical equipment measurement of earth continuity, insulation resistance, and earth leakage current are standard safety checks. If the required meters are not available I suggest a quick check with a battery and light bulb of the same low voltage to check for earth continuity.

If the machine is in working order an initial running period during which you listen and look for any abnormalities often gives an idea of what work needs to be carried out. This might be a peculiar noise, a leak (or signs of a previous leak), instability of a given measurement or a logic fault (when there is logic circuitry to control conditions in various phases of operation—for example, initial heating and subsequent cooling of a steriliser). At this stage, quick checks on calibration may point to a fault that may be dealt with easily as part of the service. Undoubtedly when you get to know a piece of equipment you develop an intuitive feel whether it is functioning normally.

Getting down to details

After the initial assessment the individual parts must be attended to. The type and amount of work required depend on the item concerned. Manufacturer's schedules should be followed, as well as any additional work suggested by the initial test run. If no information is available replace all suspect parts (when spares are available) and make good notes, labelling the various parts, to help in dismantling and reassembly. Bear in mind that most failures occur because of faults in the moving parts. A machine is composed of systems (mechanical, hydraulic, pneumatic, or electrical), and each system must be dealt with methodically and thoroughly.

Lubrication (using compatible substances) and checking of lubricant levels should be carried out frequently—for example, all the moving parts of an anaesthetic machine should be cleaned regularly and then recoated with a silicone grease. All points of contact between two surfaces, where friction is likely, should be examined for wear. If wear is noticed—for example, of gear teeth—the necessary parts may be ordered before a breakdown occurs. Catches and fastenings should be checked for secure action (for example, the port doors on incubators). Tolerances of fits should be checked; for example, slack in bearings due to wear may be evident from the measurement of the shaft diameter. This may be removed by either adjusting or replacing worn components.

Cleanliness is important, especially in dealing with hydraulic and pneumatic systems. It is essential to change or clean filters regularly, drain traps, and check tubing for deposits as well as to check all the seals. A filter is designed to stop foreign bodies travelling "downstream," so it is imperative to ensure that any debris dislodged during the cleaning of the filter or tubing is removed completely. Do not flush debris towards small orifices or low points unless these may be unblocked easily. The regular disconnection, cleaning, and reconnection of dissimilar metal components may save the aggravation of finding them seized solid; solenoid valves often suffer from this problem. All seals should be inspected for distortion; if spares are in short supply the technique of using suitable substances such as silicone grease, or the turning over of seals to use the opposite surface, may be tried.

Check and recheck

Faulty contacts are the cause of most faults in an electrical system, especially if high currents are used, and hence they should be examined frequently for damage. If the contacts are badly pitted they should be replaced; if not then any carbon deposits may be removed by rubbing fine abrasive paper between them (emery paper is not fine enough but I have used cardboard) or using contact cleaner, or both. Check that all wires are joined to the correct terminals securely, and examine the insulation of all cables. (I have encountered potentially lethal medical equipment where a castor has cut through the earth wire of a 240 V mains cable and where fuses have been bypassed by 1·25 inch nails). Check for dry solder joints; it is worth removing and cleaning all connectors as oxide layers may build up and lead to intermittent

A plain man's guide to maintenance

faults (a technician's nightmare). In extremes of humidity or when spillage is possible corrosion of copper may be prevented by varnishing or greasing. Electronic components are usually reliable, but thermionic valves, semiconductors, and polarised (marked + and −) capacitors tend to fail. It is, therefore, a good idea to replace all such components in a predetermined fault area when repairing old equipment. Dummy transducer components (often a resistor) may be used to define whether a fault is part of the electrical system or not.

Machines should be calibrated at regular intervals, and certainly after part of a system has been replaced. Measurements should be compared with measurements obtained with the most accurately known reliable instrument of the same range. Calibration should be carried out in as near normal working conditions as possible; measurements should ideally be made after a suitable warm up period followed by a soak test. In this test the machine is left running for a duration similar to that which it is used for normally. All the variables should then be re-checked. If the machine has control times and logic, these should also be checked after any final adjustments have been made.

When the routine work and subsequent testing have been completed the machine should prove to be more reliable and have a longer working life—a theory that may be compared with the treatment of patients by preventive medicine rather than cure.

Established in 1966, the Joint Mission Hospital Equipment Board was set up to coordinate and supply the medical equipment needs of mission and charity hospitals in developing countries. It was registered as an independent charity and the trading name of ECHO (equipment for charity hospitals overseas) was adopted, symbolising the widening role of the organisation. ECHO's services consist of a medical equipment service, a pharmaceutical service, an agency service for charity hospitals and grant making organisations, a specialised packing and shipping service, a veterinary division and a technical department headed by the author. Their address is ECHO, 4 West Street, Ewell, Surrey, tel 01-393 0021.

OBSTETRIC CARE

JILL EVERETT

Obstetric care in Third World hospitals differs from that in Britain in several important respects. Skill, drugs, equipment, and finance may be limited, and the large number of patients cared for may make overcrowding a serious problem. Although the emphasis of medical care must be on prevention, complications from neglect, such as obstructed labour and ruptured uterus, are common. In addition, it is important to respect the local cultural practices and customs, and this may lead to modifications in management.

Some obstetric complications—for example, eclampsia, disproportion, and severe anaemias—are more common in certain geographical areas than in others. Thus priorities in care must focus on the local problems of the community. Certain equipment, such as a sphygmomanometer and a fetal stethoscope, is essential wherever one is practising, but other equipment and, more especially, drugs may be necessary in some areas and not in others. In addition, modifications may have to be made to fit in with the availability of drugs in different countries.

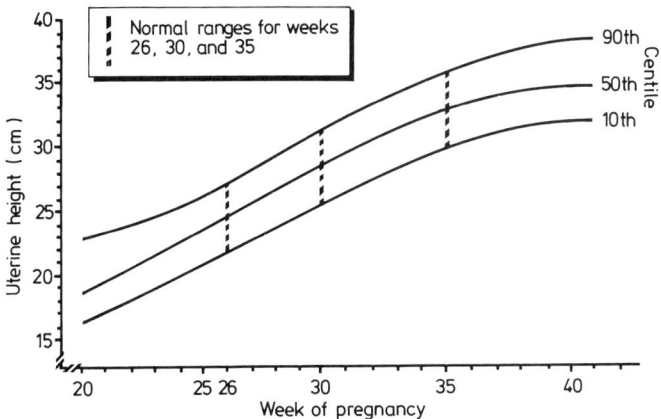

FIG 1—Graph of symphysis-fundal height, showing normal ranges of uterine height, in centimetres, by week of gestation.

The antenatal clinic

A suitable antenatal card, emphasising the detection of risk factors, is essential. Several have been designed for use in the Third World by non-medical staff,[1][2] and these may be adapted for use in hospitals.[1][2] Mothers should keep their own antenatal cards, for experience in many countries has shown that they do so safely, and it saves a great deal of time at busy clinics. In areas where intrauterine growth retardation is common a graph of symphysis-fundal height should be included in the records (fig 1). This is useful in detecting small for dates babies.[3][4]

Maternal height is an important risk factor in the Third World.[5] If a conventional measure is not available it is easy to mark a wall of the clinic. Another method is to put a bar across the door into the antenatal clinic at the local "at risk" height (fig 2). Those women who do not have to stoop to enter the room may thus be readily identified and registered as at risk. It is a waste of time to weigh women at each visit, but every woman should be weighed at her first visit and those of very low weight (below about 40 kg) should be given nutritional advice and possibly food supplements.

Facilities for testing urine for protein should be available in all areas, although they may be used only to test the urine of mothers with oedema or hypertension. Screening for glycosuria is not necessary if the prevalence of diabetes in the local population is very low. The speed and simplicity of stick tests such as Albustix and Clinistix will usually outweigh their disadvantage in cost over older methods.

The blood tests that should be performed routinely in the clinic will be influenced by the locality (for example screening

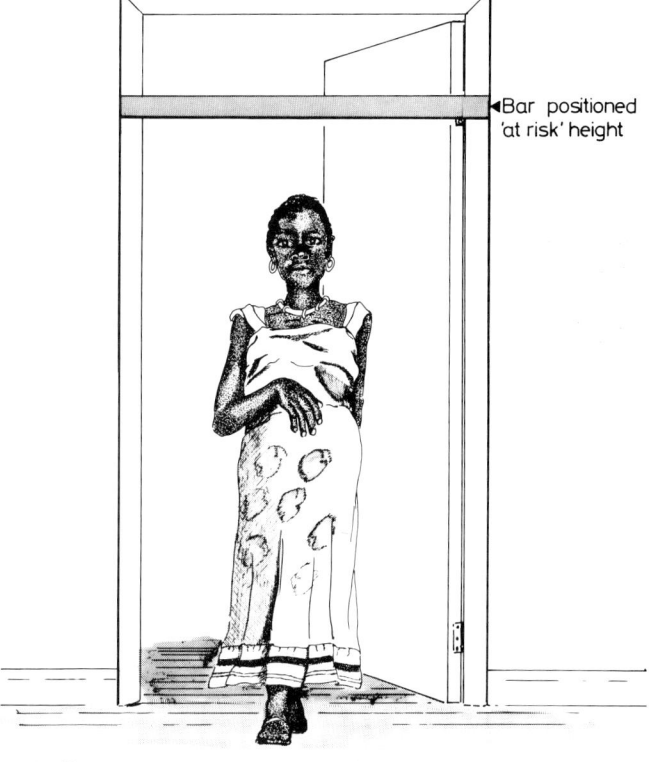

FIG 2—Bar across the door of the antenatal clinic placed at the local "at risk" height.

Obstetric care

for sickle cell disease where the population is negro), by the prevalence of diseases (serological tests for syphilis would be a high priority in Lusaka[6] but are unnecessary if syphilis is rare), and, of course, by the laboratory facilities available. The only absolutely essential blood test in all communities is the haemoglobin concentration.

Essential medication includes iron, folic acid, a simple analgesic such as soluble aspirin, and a laxative such as Senokot. Tetanus toxoid is advisable in most countries of the Third World.[7] A minimum of two doses should be given, the first as early in pregnancy as possible and the second at least two months before delivery. A booster dose should be given in subsequent pregnancies. Malarial prophylaxis is important where malaria is endemic.

The antenatal ward

This requires similar equipment to the clinic, with the following additions:

(1) Charts. A chart for recording observations on blood pressure, urine output and proteinuria, and fetal heart beat.

(2) Drugs. A local assessment should be made of the availability and cost of useful drugs. If no up to date local pharmacopoeia exists it is essential to develop your own and to work out the most cost effective treatment for a particular condition. The common obstetric problems needing drug treatment are severe

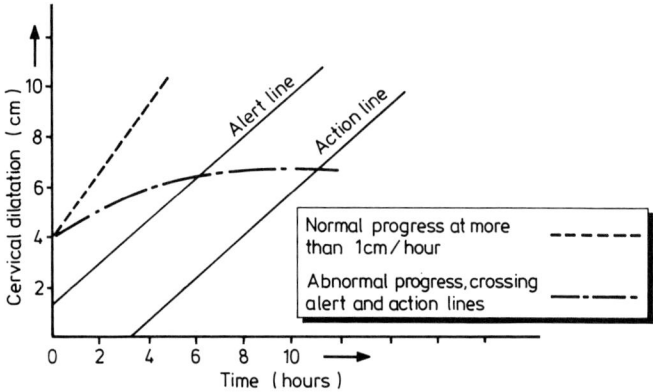

FIG 3—Partogram. The normal rate of cervical dilatation is about 1 cm/hour (the slope of the alert and action lines) The examples shown are for women found to be 4 cm dilated on admission in labour.

anaemias (sometimes with heart failure), hypertension, eclampsia, and infections. Thus a potent diuretic, quick and slow acting hypotensive agents, oral and injectable sedatives, and appropriate antibiotics must be available.

(3) Fetal monitors. The methods currently used for fetal monitoring in the United Kingdom (ultrasound measurements, tracings of fetal heart rate, and serum or urinary oestriol concentrations) are rarely practicable in Third World hospitals. Reliance should be placed on the clinical assessment of fetal growth, measurements of fundal height, and changes in maternal weight. Kick charts are suitable for literate women, in both the antenatal clinic and the ward.[8] The mother should be advised to count her baby's movements, starting at sunrise each day and stopping when she gets to ten. If she has not noticed ten movements by sunset on two successive days she should notify the midwife or doctor. A hand ultrasound fetal heart detector is useful.

Additional facilities

Referral and teaching hospitals should consider amnioscopy, which enables the forewaters to be visualised through the cervix.[9]

Assessment of volume and colour of the amniotic fluid gives an indication of fetal wellbeing. Three simple conical speculi, such as are used for fetal scalp blood sampling, together with a good light, are the only pieces of equipment required. It should also be possible to perform amniocentesis and carry out tests on the amniotic fluid. The shake test is a simplified method of assessing the lecithin:sphyngomyelin ratio and gives an estimate of lung maturity and thus of the risks of the baby developing respiratory distress after delivery.[10] Uncontaminated amniotic fluid (1 ml) is put in an 8 mm test tube. An equal volume of 95% alcohol is added and a layer of parafilm put on top, the solution is shaken vigorously for 30 seconds and then tapped to remove large bubbles. Scoring is by assessment of the foam that forms on the surface. If this forms a complete ring, the chances of respiratory distress are minimal. Gestation may be estimated by staining the fetal cells in the fluid with Nile blue sulphate; the more mature the fetus the greater the proportion of yellow staining cells.[11]

The labour ward

The labour ward must be equipped both for normal labour and delivery and for the management of all common obstetric complications and emergencies. The advantages of allowing more mobility for the woman in labour are increasingly appreciated, together with more natural positions for delivery. Some advocate the use of a simple birthing chair or stool, in addition to a standard delivery bed that must be able to tip in the head down position. An electrical or foot suction pump must be available, and even the smallest district hospital should be able to carry out an emergency caesarean section and, if possible, keep a small blood bank.

Some form of simple partogram (such as the one shown in fig 3) is essential for recording progress in labour and is invaluable in identifying early deviations from the normal. Partograms have been used successfully in many Third World countries.[13] Equipment for the management of normal labour includes a fetal stethoscope, gloves, clamps and scissors for the umbilical cord, and simple rubber or disposable catheters. Self retaining catheters should also be available for continuous bladder drainage after obstructed labour. Local anaesthesia and suturing equipment will be needed for perineal lacerations or episiotomy. Drugs must include pethidine, and ergometrine or syntometrine for use in the third stage. Syntocinon should also be available.

Every Third World labour ward should have a vacuum extractor (preferably the Bird modified Malmstrom vacuum extractor), which is a much safer and easier instrument to use than rotational forceps. There is no place for the latter unless a specialist obstetrician is present, but simple non-rotation forceps should be available. It is essential to keep adequate spare parts for the vacuum extractor, particularly chains and rubber tubing.

Operative delivery

Caesarean section is a dangerous operation in many parts of the Third World, not only because of the immediate morbidity and mortality but because of the risk of scar dehiscence in future pregnancies. In many societies abdominal delivery is regarded as a failure, and mothers may decide to go into labour at home next time, often with fatal results. Alternative management must therefore be considered, and there is a limited place for caesarean section solely in the interests of the fetus.

Symphysiotomy may have a part to play in the management of moderate disproportion. It is not a difficult operation, but doctors are strongly advised to read a detailed account before they attempt it.[14] [15] Unless the obstetrician is very experienced, symphysiotomy should be performed only in the second stage of labour and after a failed trial of vacuum extraction.

A few simple destructive instruments are necessary.[16] Perforation of the fetal head may be indicated in hydrocephaly and in obstructed labour if the cervix is fully dilated and the baby is dead. A Simpson's perforator is the best instrument, together with Willett's or Morris's forceps with which to grasp the collapsed skull. Volsellum forceps or straight clamps will do if the others are not available. A Blond Heidler saw should be kept for decapitation in an obstructed, transverse lie. It is much easier to use than a decapitation hook.

Enough general surgical instruments must be available for caesarean section, hysterectomy, and repair of a ruptured uterus to be carried out. Obtaining immediate anaesthetic care in an isolated rural hospital is usually the main problem in such cases. In the absence of a skilled anaesthetist local infiltration of the abdominal wall is a safe and satisfactory technique. More detail about anaesthesia appears in another article in this series.

Maternal complications

Haemorrhage is one of the most important causes of maternal death throughout the world, and a small blood bank with facilities for cross matching is a high priority in any hospital dealing with obstetric emergencies. Apart from saline and dextrose, a small supply of a plasma expander such as Haemaccel should be stocked.

Eclampsia is rare in Europe but still common in many parts of the Third World. A gag and airway must be present in every labour ward and stocks of an anticonvulsant, such as intravenous diazepam, should be readily available. Suitable sedative drugs such as chlorpromazine and promethazine should also be stocked.

It is not unusual for women with a haemoglobin concentration of 2-3 g/dl to walk into a Third World hospital. A blood transfusion may be life saving, but this must be carefully conducted by exchange transfusion or using packed cells and a potent diuretic such as ethacrynic acid or frusemide to avoid precipitating acute heart failure.[17] Basic equipment for exchange transfusion comprises two 50 ml syringes, two three-way taps, and the appropriate tubing.

For neonatal resuscitation a standard mouth sucker, an inclined table, readiness to give mouth to mouth respiration, and warmth are absolutely essential. Further details on this topic are given in a good account by Fawdry of low cost equipment.[18]

In this article I have not considered any expensive, modern equipment such as ultrasound scanners and electronic fetal monitoring, but if funds were available for such equipment, together with staff with the necessary skills, I would opt for a real time scanner. Its uses are wider, and it is more reliable and easier to maintain.

Fig 1 reproduced by permission from Villar J, Belizan JM, Delgado H. *Bulletin of Pan American Health Organisation* 1979;**13**, No 2:117-23.

Fig 3 reproduced by permission from Philpott RH, Castle WM. *Journal of Obstetrics and Gynaecology of the British Commonwealth* 1972;**79**:592-8.

References

[1] Dissevelt AG, Kornman JJCM, Vogel LC. An antenatal record for identification of high risk cases by auxiliary midwives at rural health centres. *Trop Geogr Med* 1976;**28**:251-5.

[2] Essex BJ, Everett VJ. Use of an action-orientated record card for antenatal screening. *Trop Doc* 1977;**7**:134-8.

[3] Belizan JM, Villar J, Nardin JC, Malamud J, Sainz de Vicuña L. Diagnosis of intrauterine growth retardation by a simple clinical method: measurement of uterine height. *Am J Obstet Gynecol* 1978;**131**:643-6.

[4] Quaranta P, Currell R, Redman CW, Robinson JS. Prediction of small for dates infants by measurement of symphysis-fundal-height. *Br J Obstet Gynaecol* 1981;**88**:115-9.

[5] Everett VJ. The relationship between maternal height and cephalopelvic disproportion in Dar es Salaam. *East Afr Med J* 1975;**52**:251-6.

[6] Watts T, Harris RR. A case-control study of stillbirths at a teaching hospital in Zambia, 1979-80: antenatal factors. *Bull WHO* 1982;**60**:971-9.

[7] Anonymous. Prevention of neonatal tetanus. *WHO Forum* 1982;**3**:432-3.

[8] Pearson JE, Weaver JB. Fetal activity and fetal well being—an evaluation. *Br Med J* 1976;**i**:1305-9.

[9] Huntingford PJ, Brunello LP, Dunstan M, et al. The technique and significance of amnioscopy. *Journal of Obstetrics and Gynaecology of the British Commonwealth* 1968;**75**:610-5.

[10] Fairbrother P, van Middelkoop A, Carson B, et al. A simple foam test on liquor amnii to predict neonatal outcome. *Trop Doct* 1979;**9**:81-4.

[11] Brosens I, Gordon H. *Journal of Obstetrics and Gynaecology of the British Commonwealth* 1966;**73**:88-90.

[12] Philpott RH, Castle WM. Cervicographs in the management of labour in primigravida. *Journal of Obstetrics and Gynaecology of the British Commonwealth* 1972;**79**:592-8.

[13] Bird GC. Cervigographic management of labour in primigravidae and multigravidae with vertex presentations. *Trop Doct* 1978;**8**:78-84.

[14] Gebbie D. Symphysiotomy. *Clin Obstet Gynecol* 1982;**9**:663-83.

[15] Kairuki HCM. The place of symphysiotomy in the treatment of disproportion in Uganda. *East Afr Med J* 1975;**52**:686-93.

[16] Lawson JB. Delivery of the dead or malformed fetus. *Clin Obstet Gynecol* 1982;**9**:745-56.

[17] Lawson JB. Severe anaemia in pregnancy, a tropical obstetric emergency. *Trop Doct* 1971;**1**:77-9.

[18] Fawdry RDS. Infant resuscitation at low cost. *Trop Doct* 1983;**13**:65-9.

Recommended reading

Obstetrics and Gynaecology in the Tropics and Developing Countries: J B Lawson and Stewart. 1967. Published by Edward Arnold.

Clin Obstet Gynecol 1982;**9**. (*Obstetric Problems in the Developing World*, ed R H Philpott.) Published by W B Saunders.

Jelliffe, D B & E F P. *Advances in International Maternal and Child Health:* D B and E F P Jelliffe. 1981, vol 1. Oxford University Press.

Maternity Services in the Developing World—What the Community Needs. Proceedings of the seventh study group of the Royal College of Obstetricians and Gynaecologists, September 1979.

CARE OF THE NEWBORN

G J EBRAHIM

The present high levels of perinatal mortality (100 per 1000 births) and maternal deaths (10 per 1000 births) in the Third World,[1-3] might be improved—not by introducing advanced medical technology, but by implementing simple common sense measures. These stem from an assessment of the factors that contribute to high risks of mortality for the mother and her infant: obstetric and medical complications, social and cultural factors, and biological determinants such as age, parity, birth interval, and nutritional state. No one factor can be taken in isolation, and because of this modern methods of obstetrics and neonatal intensive care cannot produce the appreciable and lasting benefits that accrue from a general improvement in the nutrition and health of the whole community. Improved hygiene and prenatal care, the identification of mothers at risk, and monitoring to ensure that fetal growth is adequate are essential. At present four fifths of all births in the developing world are conducted by traditional birth attendants and there is much scope for upgrading their skills through appropriate training.[4] In the Sudan a training programme was first established in 1921 and many nations have now developed similar programmes.[5-7]

Low birth weight

Low birth weight, defined as below or equal to 2500 g remains a problem in many countries (fig 1) and is one of the most important factors in the survival and well being of the infant, not only during the neonatal period but also throughout infancy. An analysis of infant mortality in Madras found that 73% of all deaths occurred in infants with birth weights of less than 2000 g.[8] The inter-American investigation of mortality in childhood found that immaturity was an underlying or associated cause of death in infancy for at least 20 per 1000 live births in several different geographical regions.[9] Thus promotion of adequate fetal growth by improving the general health and nutrition of the women in the community, especially during pregnancy, is vital. Anaemia and malnutrition must be corrected; prophylactic antimalarial treatment during the last trimester of pregnancy may also improve the weight of the infant (by as much as 160-200 g) besides conferring protection on the mother.[10]

In many communities the wet season has been identified as a particularly difficult time for pregnant and lactating women, and studies in The Gambia and Tanzania have shown the importance of seasonal influences on fetal growth, with a reduction in birth weight during the wet seasons.[11 12] This is because food stores are low at this time, and long hours of hard work on the land are needed. This work is traditionally carried out by women—irrespective of whether they are pregnant—and the increased expenditure of energy coupled with scarcity of food produces excessive nutritional demands on mothers, who may well be on the borderline of malnutrition.

Infections

Neonatal tetanus is the second most important cause of death in the newborn in developing countries and it claims more victims (over 20 per 1000 births) than the current total perinatal mortality in Britain. Effective prevention may, however, be achieved by immunising the mother with tetanus toxoid in the third trimester of pregnancy. This produces an antibody response and the antibodies cross the placenta to confer protection on the fetus. Several countries are currently setting up national strategies for preventing neonatal tetanus.[13 14]

Perinatal infection continues to be a major problem, and congenital syphilis and gonococcal ophthalmia are still encountered in the Third World. Cross infection in the newborn nursery, including eye, skin, and cord infection progressing occasionally to more generalised septicaemia, is an ever present hazard, especially when a communal bath tub or changing table is used. Mothers should be discouraged from applying anything to the cord, which is best left alone. If the child is sent home early it may be a good idea to apply the triple dye (which includes crystal violet, brilliant green, and proflavine hemisulphate) preparation as an antiseptic. Staff must be trained to provide and encourage essential measures of hygiene and basic nursing care, for such simple measures are the key to successful care of the newborn. The incidence of infection may also be reduced by encouraging breast feeding. In a recent study in the Philippines a change from routine care of the neonate in a nursery to "rooming in"—where the mother was allowed to stay permanently with the child—resulted not only in higher rates of breast feeding but also in an appreciable reduction in the incidence of sepsis and diarrhoea.[15] Another simple but important provision is that of running water, soap, and a plentiful supply of towels: this is likely to be much more effective than antibiotics for preventing sepsis. Cloth towels used by all and sundry and which remain wet most of the time are dangerous. When antibiotic treatment is indicated, careful monitoring of the common bacteria and their sensitivities may help in planning appropriate treatment.

Care of the newborn

At birth the baby's basic needs are to establish respiration and adequate nutrition, maintain normal body temperature, and avoid contact with infection. The object of care at birth is to ensure that these needs are met and to help the baby in making the adjustment to extrauterine life. Many of the diseases of the neonatal period arise from a failure to make this adjustment—for example, because of congenital malformations, maternal illness, or infection, physical or biochemical injury, or sepsis. Nevertheless, many problems are generated because of a failure to carry out routine normal procedures after the birth of healthy infants.

Care of the newborn

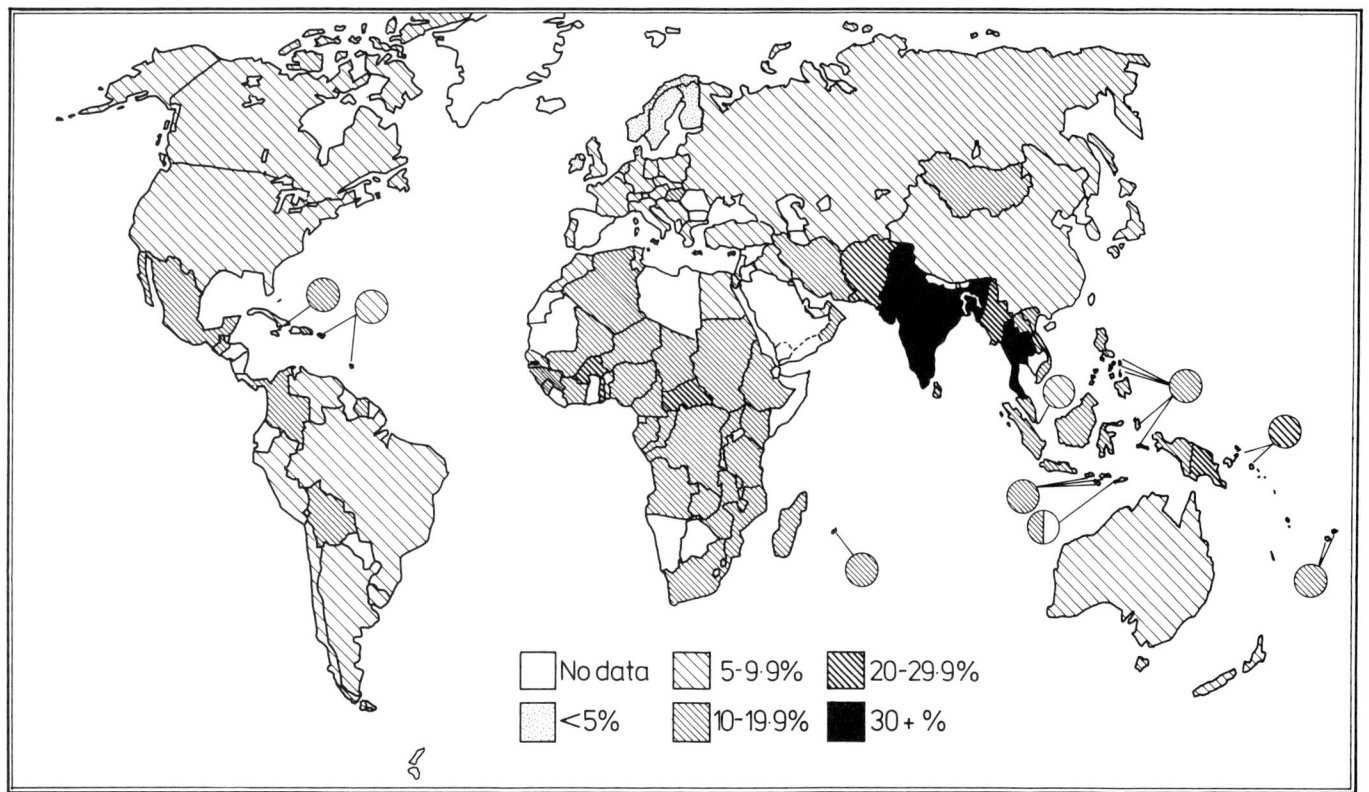

FIG 1—Prevalence of infants with low birth weight by country in 1982. (Modified from the World Health Organisation Thirty-Seventh World Health Assembly. Provisional agenda item 20, 23 March 1984.)

The most important first step after delivery is to establish respiration, and if clearing of air passages is necessary, gravity may help to drain the fluid and blood from the mouth, nose, and oropharynx. Excess mucus in the nose and mouth should be cleared with a mucus extractor, but suction must be gentle and applied briefly. Mucus extractors can be easily assembled using a 20 ml or 50 ml injection phial. Mechanical suckers in the newborn may be dangerous and are best avoided.

Apgar score

	0	1	2
Heart rate	Absent	<100/min	>100/min
Respiratory effort	Absent	Slow, regular	Good cry
Muscle tone	Limp	Some flexion of extremities	Active motion
Reflex irritability	No response	Some motion	Cry
Colour	Blue or pale	Body pink, limbs blue	Completely pink

The newborn child should be carefully examined for the presence of any obvious congenital defects or deformities. In many traditional societies abnormal babies are considered to be "bad omens" and are at risk of being neglected or even abandoned by their parents. The most widely used method to assess the vitality of the newborn is the Apgar score taken at birth and at five minutes (table). A score below 5 means that prompt action is necessary. Certain symptoms indicate serious illness, and the nursing staff should be trained to look out for such danger signals as cyanosis, pallor, bleeding, melaena, echymoses, jaundice, convulsions, no bowel movement in first 24 hours, no urine passed in first 24 hours, apnoeic spells and respiratory difficulties, vomiting, excessive drooling, inability to feed, sclerema, and oedema.

Certain obstetric situations are commonly associated with difficulty in establishing respiration and should alert the doctor to the possible need for resuscitation. These include prolonged second stage of labour, prolonged rupture of membranes, prolapse of the cord or cord entanglement, and difficulty with delivery of the shoulders. Signs of fetal distress—meconium stained liquor and changes in heart rate (tachycardia >160/min or bradycardia of <100/min) should also prompt anticipatory action.

Resuscitation

The basic principles of resuscitation of a baby who is not breathing are as follows:

(1) Establish and maintain airway through suction and insertion of an airway.

(2) Ensure oxygenation (at a flow rate of 4 litres/min if administered by a funnel and 1 litre/min if via a nasal catheter).

(3) Secure adequate ventilation by mouth to mouth respiration (rate 40/min) while occluding the oesophagus with finger pressure over the cricoid, or by Ambu bag and mask if available.

(4) Correct acidosis if necessary (intravenous sodium bicarbonate 3 ml/kg of an 8·4% solution).

(5) Support circulation by cardiac massage if necessary (rate 80-100 per minute).

Stimulation of the respiratory centre by analeptics (for example, nikethamide) is unnecessary and may be dangerous. If the mother has had pethidine then naloxone hydrochloride (60 micrograms/kg) by intramuscular injection is helpful. Infants who have difficulty establishing respiration will usually have difficulty in

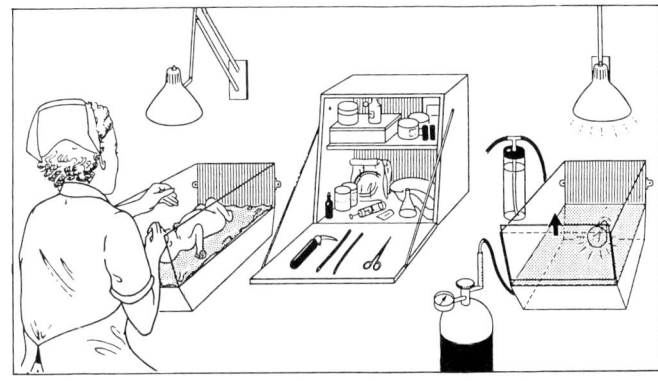

FIG 2—Equipment for care of the newborn. (Modified from the Teaching Aids at Low Cost (TALC) set of teaching slides on care of the newborn.)

Care of the newborn

maintaining it; hence careful observation for a day or so is necessary. An apnoea alarm may be valuable in alerting the staff to take prompt action. The Draeger apnoea alarm is reliable and sturdy and requires little servicing. It costs about £150 and the pads, which need to be changed regularly, are £26 each. Apnoeic spells (pauses greater than 20 seconds) or the development of a dusky colour due to poor respiratory drive often respond to theophylline 2 mg/kg every eight hours. Other causes of apnoea —for example, intracranial bleeding, patent ductus arteriosus, pneumonia, sepsis, and the respiratory distress syndrome—should be carefully looked for. If aspiration of meconium has occurred tracheal intubation and careful sucking out are necessary. A good infant laryngoscope with a MacIntosh or straight blade is essential, together with endotracheal tubes of sizes 2·5 to 5 mm.

Neonatal intensive care

The major debate in centres providing neonatal care is on the cost and effectiveness of neonatal intensive care units. It is estimated that in the United States it costs about $1000 a day for a baby to be in intensive care, and the average stay is 23 days. The care of very small infants (<1000 g) costs proportionately more.[16] Nevertheless, a neonatal unit need not be expensive, and in my view a district hospital in the Third World should have a newborn unit to provide special care for those babies that require it. The unit may also be of value for training and counselling health care workers on how to care for the newborn and how to establish and supervise simple common sense routines for handling babies who have special problems.

Improved mortality figures in the West stem from the prevention and treatment of birth asphyxia, birth trauma, hypothermia, hypoglycaemia, and hyperbilirubinaemia. Both hypoglycaemia and hyperbilirubinaemia may be prevented by early feeding with breast milk, which is now routine in many neonatal units.[17] Dextrostix provide a simple way to diagnose hypoglycaemia and they should be kept in all neonatal units. (In tropical climates it is important to store them in a cool place; otherwise their life is limited.) Deaths in infants weighing 1500 g or less may be reduced by about a quarter if their body temperature is maintained above 36°C and heat loss is kept at a minimum.[18] The infant is particularly vulnerable at the time of delivery because of a sudden drop in environmental temperature and evaporative heat loss from a wet skin. What is tolerably warm for an adult may still be too cold for a small newborn baby. Immediate drying of the wet skin, adequate covering, including the head, and nursing close to the mother's body for warmth should prevent hypothermia in most cases, but if the infant's body temperature does drop bottles of warm water, radiant heaters, or even an Anglepoise lamp may help. Hypothermia is easily dealt with provided it is diagnosed promptly. A low reading rectal thermometer should be available in all neonatal units. In many Third World countries the ambient temperature is such that only minimal heating is required to keep the temperature at a satisfactory level, so most neonatal units will not need incubators, which are expensive and need frequent servicing.

Incubators should thus be reserved for those babies who are very ill or who must be nursed naked for continuous monitoring. The choice of incubator should be guided by the facilities that it offers: the best ones have a side opening, good air circulation, thermostatically controlled heat regulation, and provision for cooling by ice if necessary, and they are easy to disinfect after use. Incubators which offer too many elaborations and need frequent servicing are best avoided. The Vickers incubator is good but costs £2900 and needs regular servicing, so its use will be restricted to those teaching hospitals and referral centres which can afford it. Figure 2 illustrates the equipment that is needed for care of the newborn.

Problems in the first week

Pulmonary immaturity and ventricular haemorrhage are the leading causes of death in preterm babies during the first week of life. The hallmark of good respiratory care in the newborn is prompt intervention before the infant's condition deteriorates to a state where full ventilatory support is necessary. Much of the improvement in neonatal mortality in the developed countries stems from prompt and effective management of asphyxia rather than from the treatment of respiratory distress syndrome.[19] The danger signals are delayed onset of respiration at birth, recurrent apnoeic episodes, tachypnoea of more than 50/min in the second hour of life, and hypothermia. The principles to adopt are well established[20]: (a) prompt and efficient resuscitation of the preterm infant to establish ventilation and to help release surfactant from the pneumocytes; (b) avoidance of hypothermia, hypoxia, and acidaemia because of their secondary effects on the synthesis of surfactant.

Any unit undertaking mechanical ventilation for the respiratory distress syndrome must have an adequate number of trained nurses, staff skilled in arterial catheterisation and administering intravenous therapy, and a reliable laboratory to carry out essential biochemical tests. In the absence of these facilities there is little point in trying to run a neonatal intensive care unit.

Several specific problems occur in certain geographical areas. G6PD deficiency as a cause of neonatal jaundice is often encountered, especially among the Chinese, in west Africa, in some Mediterranean countries, and in some ethnic groups in South East Asia. Prophylactic phototherapy is an effective way to treat neonatal jaundice if the rise in serum bilirubin concentration is gradual. A simple icterometer may help in early selection of babies who need phototherapy, and a canopy using fluorescent lamps is easy to assemble. (It is worth remembering that an infant in an incubator near a window who is exposed to six hours of daylight receives more of the effective wave length than an infant under a light canopy for 24 hours.)

Conclusion

Programmes of care for the newborn in the developing world must focus on the problem of low birth weight, for up to a third of all newborn infants fall into this group—most of them because of inadequate growth in fetal life. Priority should be given to prevention, which may be achieved through adequate prenatal care. A knowledge of neonatal physiology and the prompt instigation of immediate care of the small infant are essential, for thorough assessment and routine treatment may do much to reduce neonatal morbidity and mortality.[21]

References

1 World Health Organisation. *The prevention of perinatal morbidity and mortality.* Geneva: WHO, 1981.
2 World Health Organisation. *Maternal mortality. World health statistics report.* Vol 30, No 4. Geneva: WHO, 1977.
3 Barns TEC. Obstetrics in the third world with particular reference to field research into delivery of maternal care to the community. In: Stallworthy J, Bourne G, eds. *Recent advances in obstetrics and gynaecology.* London: Churchill Livingstone, 1979:109-36. (No 13.)
4 Anonymous. Why retain traditional birth attendants? *Lancet* 1983;i:223-4.
5 Mangay-Maglacas A, Pizurki H, eds. *The traditional birth attendant in seven countries: case studies in utilisation and training.* Geneva: WHO, 1981.
6 Bella H, Ebrahim GJ. The village midwives of the Sudan. An enquiry into the availability and quality of maternity care. *J Trop Ped* 1984;30:115-8.
7 Verderese M de L, Turnbull LM. *The traditional birth attendant in maternal and child health and family planning.* Geneva: WHO, 1974.
8 Gopalan C. Effect of nutrition on pregnancy and lactation. *Bull WHO* 1962;26:203.
9 Puffer RR, Serrano CV. *Patterns of mortality in childhood.* Washington DC: Pan American Health Organization, 1973:81-90.
10 McGregor JD, Avery JG. Malaria transmission and foetal growth. *Br Med J* 1974;iii:433-6.
11 Rowland MGM, Paul A, Prentice AM, *et al.* Seasonability and the growth of infants in a Gambian village. In: Chambers R, Longhurst R, Pavey A, eds. *Seasonal dimensions to rural poverty.* London: Francis Pinter, 1981:164-74.
12 Bantje H. Seasonal variations in birth weight distribution in Ikwiriri Village, Tanzania. *J Trop Ped* 1983;29:50-4.
13 World Health Organisation. Expanded programme of immunisation. Prevention of neonatal tetanus. *Weekly Epidemiological Record* 1982;No 18:127-42.
14 Anonymous. Prevention of neonatal tetanus. *Lancet* 1983;i:1253-4.
15 Clavano NR, Mode of feeding and its effect on infant mortality and morbidity. *J Trop Ped* 1982;28:287-93.
16 Pomerance JJ, Ukrainski CT, Ukso T, *et al.* Cost of living for infants weighing 1000 g or less at birth. *Pediatrics* 1980;61:908-10.
17 Davies PA, Russell H. Later progress of 100 infants weighing 1000 to 2000 g at birth fed immediately with breast milk. *Dev Med Ch Neur* 1968;10:725-35.
18 Hey EN. Thermal regulation in the newborn. *Br J Hosp Med* 1972;8:51-64.
19 Barron AJ, Tasker M, Lieberman EF, Hellier VF. Impact of improved perinatal care on the causes of death. *Arch Dis Child* 1984;59:199-207.
20 Robertson NRC. Developments in neonatal pediatric practice. In: Hull D, ed. *Recent advances in paediatrics—6.* London and Edinburgh: Churchill Livingstone, 1981:17.
21 Care of the newborn. Slide series from Teaching Aids at Low Cost, PO Box 219, St Albans, Herts AL1 4AX.

CHILD HEALTH

G J EBRAHIM

Much of the mortality and morbidity among children in developing countries is preventable. The three main causes of admissions to hospital are protein energy malnutrition, respiratory infections, and diarrhoea. These three account for 30-40% of all paediatric admissions. The next most common illnesses are anaemia, common infections of childhood such as measles and pertussis, parasitic diseases (especially malaria and intestinal helminths), tuberculosis, and burns and other accidents including poisoning. Together these nine conditions account for most of the paediatric problems in the developing world.

Undernutrition and infection make a lethal combination

Nutritional surveys of preschool children have shown that about half the children in the poorer communities are undernourished. These children have a low resistance to infection, and each minor illness tends to run a protracted course, which results in further deterioration of the children's nutritional state. Multiple pathological conditions may coexist, and many of the children who are admitted to hospital with protein energy malnutrition have other medical problems such as anaemia, vitamin deficiencies, and lower respiratory tract infections including tuberculosis. For these children even a trivial illness may precipitate a life threatening condition.

The extent to which poor nutrition influences mortality is shown in a study of 3000 children aged 1-36 months in the Punjab. Child mortality doubled with each 10% decline in body weight below 80% of the Harvard median.[1] A similar study in Bangladesh showed that children who weighed less than 65% of the Harvard median had a threefold higher death rate in the next two years compared with those whose weights were above this level; the 10% of children with the smallest arm circumference had a five times higher risk of death than the top 10%.[2]

Providing preventive services

Preventive services are important in the developing countries, where the high infant and child mortality is due not to exotic "tropical" diseases but to diseases that result from poverty, ignorance, and neglect. In order to come to grips with the determinants of disease the health professionals must feel responsible not only for those who seek their help in the hospitals but also for those who do not or cannot. Personal services such as under 5s clinics, prenatal care, and maternity care are particularly important. Preventive care does, however, require painstaking skills of gathering data, organisation, and management. The district hospital should promote this care and get the local community to participate fully in the planning, implementation, and evaluation of health care policies. The hospital also has an educative role in training health staff, who need to have adequate communication, epidemiological, and management skills to run the preventive clinics effectively. Appropriate technology is not about devices only. It also takes into account the organisational, managerial, and educational aspects of community health services. All the resources of the community need to be mobilised to create awareness and interest in health and nutrition. The schools are an important resource, which has remained untapped. The child-to-child programme, which aims at training primary school children in providing better care to their siblings at home, is an example of innovative health education.

The routine activities of the under 5s clinic include surveillance of growth by regular weighing or measurement of arm circumference. Parents may not know exactly how old their children are, but arm circumference changes little between the ages of 1 and 5, so that this measurement is a good way of identifying malnourished children. The tape may be made from an old x ray film, which is cheap and does not stretch. This should be cleaned to remove the gelatine, and then a strip may be marked off as shown (fig 1). The tape may be coloured to make the measurements easy to interpret. Any child whose arm circumference is below 12·5 cm—that is, in the red zone—is considered to be malnourished; 12·5-13·5 cm is borderline; and above 13·5 cm the child is adequately nourished. Monitoring the

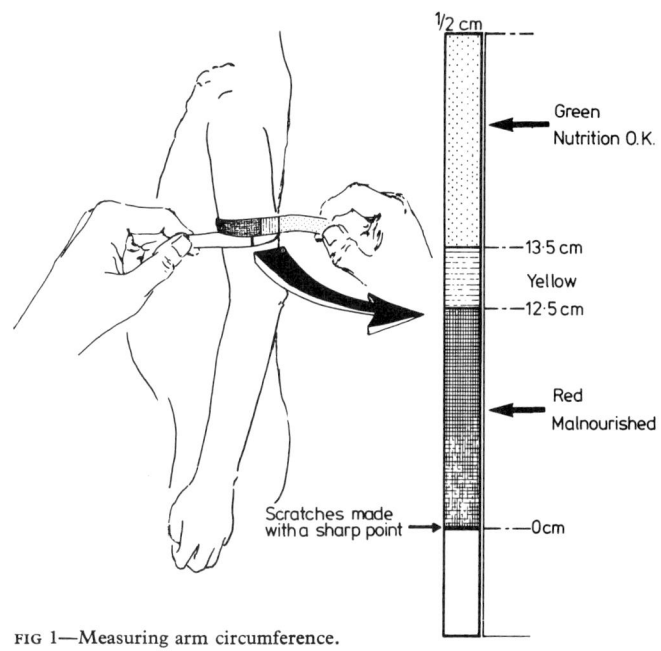

FIG 1—Measuring arm circumference.

Child health

rate of growth in childhood is important, for growth is a sensitive indicator not only of health and nutritional state but also of illnesses and even emotional upsets. Thus growth charts should be kept, and the shape of a child's growth curve is a sensitive indicator of his wellbeing. The growth chart shown in fig 2 is adapted from the one currently recommended by the World Health Organisation and the United Nations Children's Fund. Local growth standards vary from country to country, but the World Health Organisation has issued a growth chart for international use based on growth data for children in the United States.[3]

In addition to surveillance of growth, under 5s clinics provide an immunisation service and advise mothers on infant feeding and family planning. The clinics may also have a diagnostic role and give advice and treatment for common disorders such as diarrhoea, malnutrition, and intestinal infestation. Experience in several countries has shown that the under 5s clinics (and the antenatal and maternal clinics) may be run by auxiliary health workers provided they have periodic supervision and back up from professional health staff.

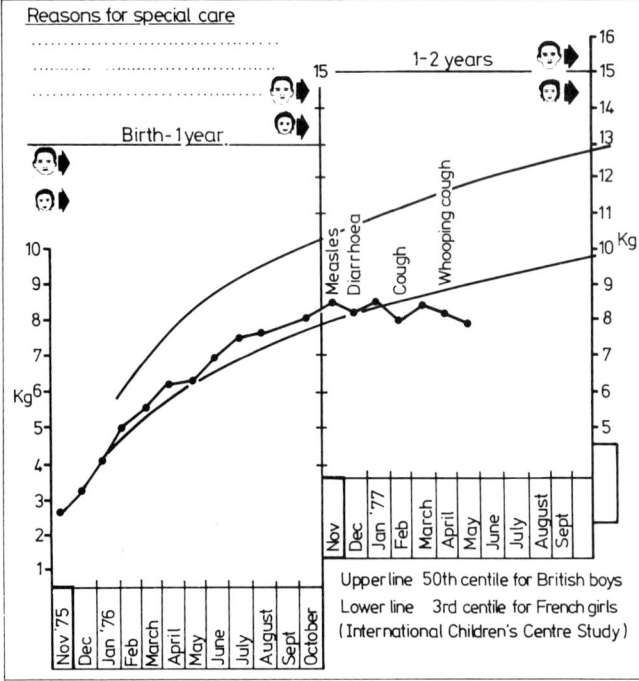

FIG 2—Growth chart, suitable for both boys and girls.

Under 5s clinics perform two important functions besides their purely medical ones. They can become the springboards for a number of community activities. As such they have an important supportive role towards other community health workers. Secondly, they can identify individuals and families at risk for more intensive care and counselling. If the coverage by the maternal and child health services is adequate regular collection of data may yield valuable information for developing criteria for identifying those at risk of diseases among the local community. This is important as it enables the community to identify the preventable antecedents of malnutrition and other illnesses and offers the opportunity to provide appropriate health education and early corrective action.[4]

Developments in child care

Three recent developments in nutritional and medical care hold promise for the future: firstly, a better understanding of the nutritional requirements of children and of the pathophysiology and management of diarrhoea; secondly, improved immunisation policies and methods and new, more robust vaccines; and, thirdly, advances in the intermediate technology for providing safe water and disposal of waste. These three factors have prompted the World Health Organisation and the United Nations Children's Fund to promote new strategies and health programmes.[3] These include an expanded programme of immunisation and the promotion of oral rehydration therapy. These aim at helping developing countries achieve better levels of immunisation than the previous 11-20% and setting up nationwide facilities for the management of diarrhoea. (These programmes also include strategies for training health workers, methods of epidemiological surveillance, and the development of facilities for storage and transport of necessary supplies.)

Nutrition

Mother's milk is now recognised to be the sheet anchor of sound infant and child nutrition,[5 6] as well as contributing to mother-infant bonding. Human milk contains only 1% protein (range 9·5-12·0 g/l),[7] but at 25 J (6 cal)/g solid matter human milk has one of the highest energy densities among foods, and infants all over the world thrive on it, doubling their weights during the first four months of life when fed on breast milk alone. The origins of malnutrition are often traced to the weaning period with the introduction of local staple foods in the form of a gruel.[8] Many traditional gruels have an energy density of only 4·2 J (1 cal)/g, and the sudden change from an energy rich food to a watery gruel is largely responsible for the slowing of growth. Hence the emphasis in nutritional education has shifted from the concentration of protein to the energy content of weaning foods.

The main problem with traditional gruels is the high starch content, the source of energy in all cereals and tubers. On heating in water starch granules swell and coalesce, resulting in increased viscosity, which increases even further on cooling.[9] The young infant can manage only foods of a fluid consistency, so there is a limit to the amount of cereal that can be used in the preparation of the gruels, most of which contain 85-90% water. One way out of the dilemma is to add a small quantity of edible oil to the gruel. This not only increases the energy content but also helps to keep the consistency of the gruel more fluid. Similar considerations apply to solid foods. For example, boiled rice is up to 65% water; if foods containing fat, such as ground nut, soya, or coconut, are added this increases the energy content. Alternatively, if the cereal grain is sprouted before it is ground into flour the amount of starch is reduced by conversion to dextrins, dextrimaltose, and maltose, and so much more flour can be added to make a gruel of the same viscosity.

Adequate amounts of essential amino acids in the weaning diet may be provided by a judicious mixture of cereals and legumes.[10] Cereals tend to be low in lysine content but relatively rich in amino acids containing sulphur. Regional recipes for weaning foods based on multimixes have been developed for most countries.[11]

Oral rehydration: a major breakthrough

Oral rehydration, with a sugar and electrolyte solution, for the management of diarrhoea in children has led to an improvement in mortality as well as early recovery.[12] The mixture currently recommended for oral rehydration[13] contains glucose 110 mmol/l (2·0 g/100 ml) (made from 20 g glucose); sodium 90 mmol (mEq)/l (3·5 g sodium chloride); potassium 20 mmol (mEq)/l (1·5 g potassium chloride); chloride 80 mmol (mEq)/l (2·5 g sodium bicarbonate); and bicarbonate 30 mmol (mEq)/l (1 l water).

The distribution and provision of a continuous supply of prepackaged ingredients are unlikely to be practicable for every

Child health

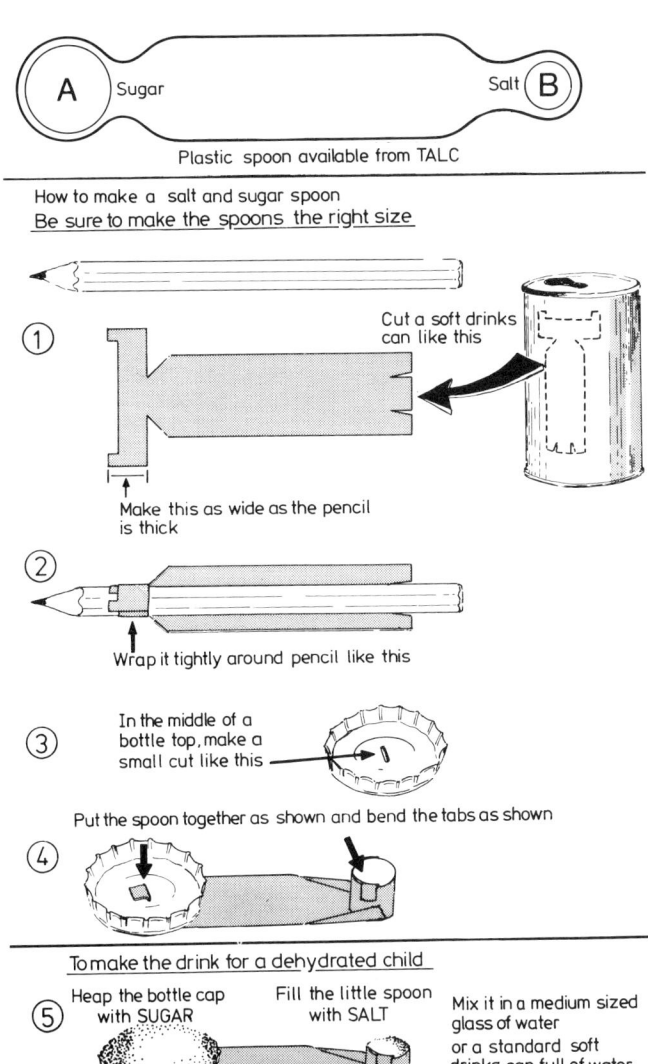

FIG 3—Plastic spoon used in making up a simple oral rehydration fluid, and the do it yourself equivalent.

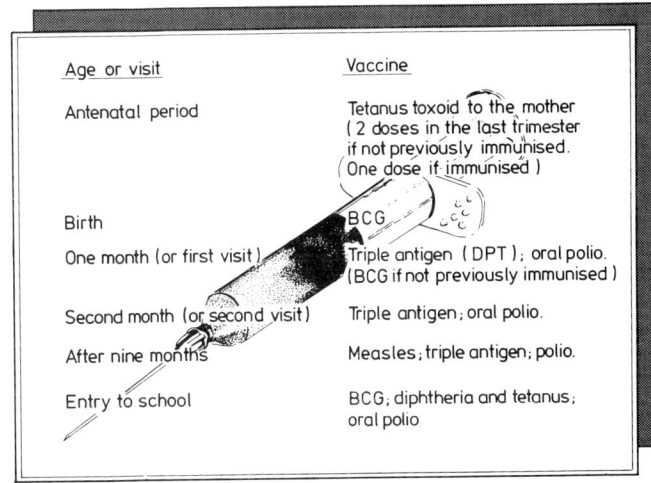

FIG 4—Recommended schedule of immunisation.

village and settlement, but the techniques may be simplified. Mothers should be shown how to make the solution from sugar, salt, and water, using a special plastic spoon (available from TALC, PO Box 49, St Albans, Herts) or a home made scoop (fig 3). The solution should be freshly made up each time, for it supports bacterial growth and may easily become contaminated if left to stand for long periods. One large scoop of cane sugar and one small scoop of salt should be added to a glass or cupful (200 ml) of boiled clean water. The child should be given one cupful for each bowel movement during the episode of diarrhoea. Breast feeding should continue, and the older infant should be persuaded to eat a normal diet, for he or she is likely to absorb about 70% of the nutrient value of the food despite the diarrhoea. An alternative to the sugar and salt solution is to give the child the water that the family boils the rice in. This contains salt and starch and is an effective form of fluid replacement for the dehydrated child.

Immunisation

The role of immunisation in controlling the prevalence of pertussis, diphtheria, poliomyelitis, and measles is well known. The success of relatively poor countries such as Cuba, China, and Sri Lanka in achieving high rates of immunisation has shown that it is not the cost of vaccines but the ability and determination to set up a delivery system that are the crucial factors. Preventive services such as the under 5s clinic should carry out immunisation, and the standard schedule that is applicable to all Third World countries is shown in fig 4. Successful uptake rates with live polio vaccine have been low in some countries—about 50%, compared with about 90% in Western countries. Possibly the cluster technique of immunisation, whereby many children are offered the vaccine on the same day, may help improve these low conversion rates.[13] (The value of BCG is under question, but the World Health Organisation recommends the continued use of vaccine that is currently available until further information is accrued.[14])

In all developing countries that have made rapid progress in health the key factors have been community awareness and good organisation, and these have enabled the local preventive service programmes to be implemented.

The illustrations were adapted from *Paediatric Practice in Developing Countries*, by G J Ebrahim.

References

[1] Kielman AA, McCord C. Weight for age as an index of risk of death in children. *Lancet* 1978;i:1247-50.
[2] Chen LC, Chowdhuryt AKMA, Huttman SL. Anthropometric assessment of energy protein malnutrition and subsequent risk of mortality among pre-school age children. *Am J Clin Nutr* 1980;**33**:1836-45.
[3] World Health Organisation. *A growth chart for international use in maternal and child health care. Guidelines for primary health care personnel.* Geneva: WHO, 1978.
[4] Al-Dabagh A, Ebrahim GJ. The preventable antecedents of childhood malnutrition. *J Trop Pediatr* 1984;**30**:50-2.
[5] Ebrahim GJ. *Breastfeeding, the biological option.* London: Macmillan Press, 1978.
[6] Jelliffe DB, Jelliffe EPP. *Human milk in the modern world.* Oxford: Oxford University Press, 1978.
[7] Department of Health and Social Security. *The composition of human milk.* London: HMSO, 1977. (Report on Health and Social Subjects No 12.)
[8] Rutishauser IHE. Growth of the pre-school child in West Mengo district, Uganda. In: Ower R, Ongom VL, Kirya BC, eds. *The child in the African environment—growth, development and survival.* Nairobi: East African Literature Bureau, 1974.
[9] Ljungquist BG, Mellander O, Svanberg US. Dietary bulk as a limiting factor for nutritional intake in pre-school children. *J Trop Pediatr* 1981;**27**:68-73.
[10] Protein Advisory Group. *Guidelines on protein food mixtures for older infants and young children.* New York: United Nations, 1970. (Guideline No 8.)
[11] Cameron M, Hofvander Y. *Manual on feeding infants and young children.* Oxford: Oxford University Press, 1983.
[12] International Study Group. Beneficial effects of oral electrolyte-sugar solutions in the treatment of children's diarrhoea. Studies in seven rural villages. *J Trop Pediatr* 1981;**27**:136-9.
[13] John TJ, Joseph A, Vijayarethnam P. A better system for polio vaccination in developing countries. *Br Med J* 1980;**281**:542.

Child health

[14] World Health Organisation. *Treatment and prevention of dehydration in diarrhoeal diseases: a guide for use at the primary level.* Geneva: WHO, 1976.

Recommended reading

Nutrition for Developing Countries: M King, D Morley, L and A Burgess. Written in simple English, with exercises that can be undertaken in the community (English Language Book Society edition.)

Using the Method of Paulo Freire in Nutrition Education: Therese Drummond. Excellent account of adult literacy and nutrition programme.

Paediatric Priorities in the Developing World: David Morley. Alternative priorities to those suggested by traditional paediatrics. (English Language Book Society edition, Indonesian, Spanish, Portuguese, or French.)

See How They Grow: David Morley. A follow on to *Paediatric Priorities in the Developing World:* the importance of the growth chart is emphasised. Also in Spanish.

Primary Child Care Book One: Maurice and Felicity King: Comprehensive child care in simple language, well illustrated.

Primary Child Care Book Two: A Guide for the Community Leader, Manager and Teacher: Maurice and Felicity King. An excellent and most useful book; also contains 3000 multiple choice questions.

Manual on Feeding Infants and Young Children: M Cameron and Y Hofvander. A new edition completely rewritten; simple and practical.

Child to Child. Prepared for the International Year of the Child, this describes how older children can help younger children's health and development.

Practical Mother and Child Health in Developing Countries (intended for the community nurse), *Care of the Newborn in Developing Countries* (for the midwife), *Child Care in the Tropics* (for the health educator), *Breastfeeding: the Biological Option* (for the nutrition worker), *A Handbook of Tropical Paediatrics* (for the medical auxiliary): all by G J Ebrahim from the health care centre set of books (English Language Book Society editions).

Paediatric Practice in Developing Countries: G J Ebrahim (English Language Book Society edition available).

Child Health in a Changing Environment: G J Ebrahim. Sponsored by the World Health Organisation as part of the activities of the International Year of the Child, the book is written for health planners.

Nutrition in Mother and Child Health: G J Ebrahim.

District Health Care: Challenges for Planning Organisation and Evaluation in Developing Countries: Lartson A, Ebrahim GJ, Lovel HJ, Ranken JP.

All the above titles are available from: Teaching Aids at Low Cost, Institute of Child Health, 30 Guildford Street, London WC1N 1EH.

A series of titles published by the African Medical Research Foundation, PO Box 30125, Nairobi, Kenya.

ANAESTHETICS

F N PRIOR

It is a sad fact that many doctors in countries where access to Western technology is limited regard the "rag and bottle" type of anaesthesia as all that is possible unless complicated machines are available. It is another sad fact that many trained anaesthetists also believe this and that such machines are essential to undertake major surgery. In this article I attempt to show that there is an alternative, and that anaesthetic running costs may be kept to a minimum while the scope and flexibility of Boyle's, Heidbrink, or other similar machines are retained. The approach advocated is practical and reasonable and is not offered as a second best. (Costs are indicated in current sterling prices, although most will be higher in Third World countries because of customs dues and dealers' profits.)

Local techniques are the mainstay of anaesthetic practice in many small hospitals and, indeed, should be, but for this very reason doctors tend to have more experience in their use than in general anaesthetic techniques. Several good teaching texts are available, and a selection is listed at the end of this article. Of the local anaesthetic blocks that are of most practical use, spinal blocks undoubtedly head the list. Epidurals will be possible for those who are keen on developing their use. Either technique is appropriate for most analgesic requirements in the abdomen and legs. Among the nerve blocks, brachial block by the supraclavicular or axillary approach is useful, as is Bier's block (intravenous perfusion of the limb). Field blocks of the abdominal wall are not easy to perform, but an inject and cut technique is safe and simple, especially for repair of a hernia.

Inhalational anaesthesia

Inhalational anaesthesia will be the standard method of maintaining anaesthesia for the foreseeable future. The impression gained is that this needs complicated equipment, but this is not necessarily so. Much of the apparent complexity is due to dependence on supplies of nitrous oxide and oxygen, which are stored under high pressures in cylinders. In many Third World countries distribution of these gases is likely to produce transport problems, and (even if they are available) the supply may be uncertain and the equipment, as well as the nitrous oxide, is expensive (tables I and II). It is possible, however, to give perfectly adequate and controlled anaesthesia without nitrous oxide, using relatively simple apparatus. It is desirable to have oxygen, but if this is used alone a simple flow meter with a regulator is all that is needed, and provided that the gas is used economically large stocks are not required—indeed, air alone is sufficient for most patients, and the oxygen may be kept for those who really need it.

The cost and availability of anaesthetic inhalation agents will determine what may be used, but most anaesthetists working in developing countries will have access to ether. This had a reputation for producing a prolonged hangover due to its inappropriate use,[1] but it can be used safely now that concentrations may be measured and administration easily controlled. The same applies to trichloroethylene (Trilene)[2] and halothane—also to ethrane and isoflurane, but these two are expensive and unsuitable for general use. Methoxyflurane has been withdrawn from manufacture because of renal side effects, and although it may still be offered for sale, it is best avoided. All these agents may be used for spontaneous or controlled respiration either by hand or using a ventilator.[3 4] Table I summarises

TABLE I—*Cost of anaesthetic drugs*

Agent	Ventilating concentrations Controlled	Ventilating concentrations Spontaneous	Rough cost/hour	Comments
Ether	2-3%	6-8%	12-50p	At low concentrations no more vomiting than with nitrous oxide. Not explosive in air
Trichloroethylene	0·3-0·5%	Not suitable	3p	Good postoperative pain relief
Halothane	0-0·5%	1-2·5%	30-70p	Poor analgesia. Good induction agent. Useful in combination with trichloroethylene
Nitrous oxide	5 litres/min		80p	Transport, regulators, etc, extra

TABLE II—*Equipment costs*

Equipment	Cost (£)	Comments
EMO with bellows and connections	711	A complete set up but much improved with OMV
Bellows alone	150	Usually cheaper if made locally
OMV vapouriser alone	225	
Cyprane draw over vapouriser	440	
Boyle's without accessories	3775	
Cylinders if not available for rent (12 each for nitrous oxide and oxygen)	1248	Expect hold ups in supply. Oxygen often available locally in rented cylinders. Danger of lethal contaminants in nitrous oxide
East Radcliffe positive pressure ventilator:		
Battery or mains	1595	Uses 12 volt car battery
Mains only	700	May be supplied for 110 or 220 V
Oxford ventilator Mk 1	1865	Driven by separate supply of oxygen or compressed air: not practical unless these are freely available
Oxygen concentrator (Drager)	1500	Not yet fully tested in field conditions and servicing may be a problem

Anaesthetics

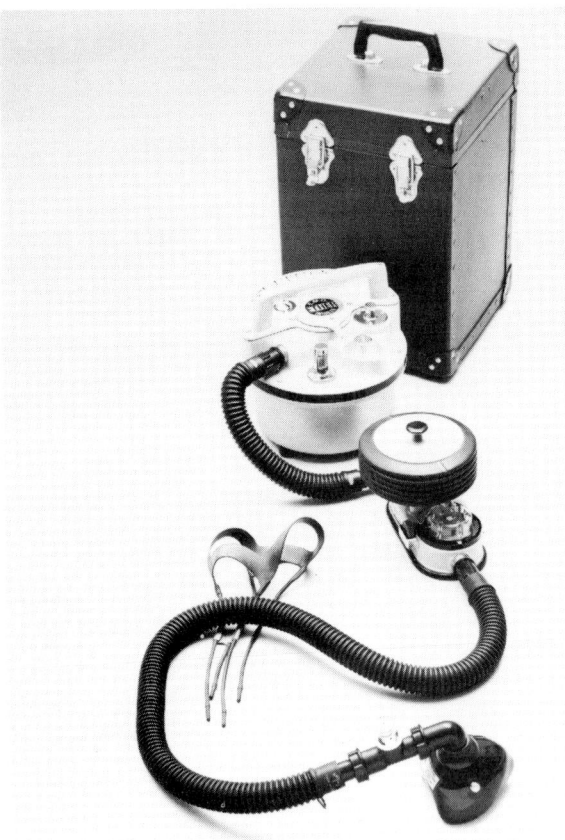

FIG 1—EMO with accessories set up for use in spontaneous respiration.

some facts about these agents together with their costs on an hourly basis; nitrous oxide is included for comparison. It should be noted that ether is explosive only if mixed with oxygen and is inflammable at a concentration of $\geqslant 1\cdot5\%$ in air, so diathermy and endoscopy should be avoided when it is in use.

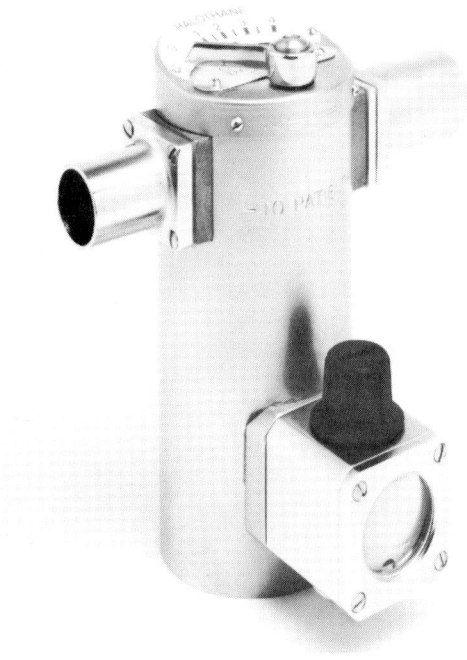

FIG 2—OMV. This can be obtained with either right to left or left to right gas flow.

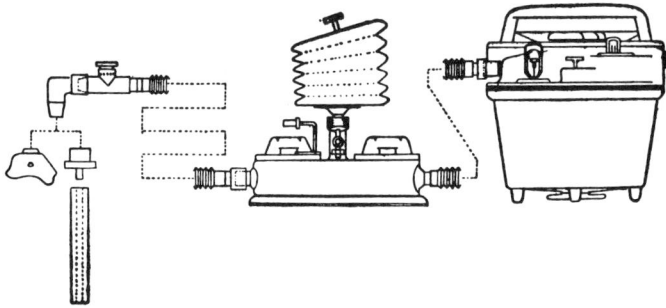

FIG 3—Diagram of possible arrangements of a draw over system. An OMV, Cyprane, or locally made vapouriser may be substituted for the EMO and a ventilator, which can be used as a draw over, for the bellows. The expiratory valve is for spontaneous respiration only. In controlled ventilation a non-rebreathing valve must be used, in which the return valve in the bellows, closest to the patient, must be immobilised. A magnet is provided for this.

Equipment

To be effective anaesthetic equipment must meet certain requirements:

(1) Afford reliable control of anaesthetic concentrations.
(2) Use atmospheric air as a vapourising agent.
(3) Permit enrichment of air with oxygen.
(4) Spontaneous or controlled respiration must be possible.
(5) The equipment may be used with a ventilator.

All these conditions are met by two anaesthetic machines—namely, the EMO (Epstein, Macintosh, Oxford) and the OMV (Oxford Miniature Vaporiser)—both of which act as draw over vaporisers. This means that the inspiratory phase of respiration produced by the patient will draw air and, if needed, oxygen through the vaporiser at a set concentration. A bellows or self inflating bag is included in the system to allow gas to flow in one way only and this leads to an expiratory valve or a non-rebreathing valve that makes artificial ventilation easy. The exhaled gas passes out of the system completely (see figs 1, 2, and 3). As an alternative, a similar draw over apparatus is made by Cyprane and an Ambu type bag may be used instead of the bellows.

All the vaporisers give reliable concentrations of gas and air, which are constant in different conditions of flow and temperature. Detailed information on variations is supplied by the manufacturers, which are listed at the end of this article.

Maintenance of the equipment is minimal and can be done by the anaesthetist on the spot—the manufacturers will supply the few necessary tools and detailed manuals. This is in contrast to the more complicated maintenance of a Boyle's machine, which entails calling out an expensive maintenance mechanic from the company.

The EMO is designed for use with ether only, but the OMV may be used with all volatile agents, for which alternative scales are available. Hence, flexibility is enhanced if the machines are used in tandem with two different agents, such as halothane and trichloroethylene. Locally made, non-thermocompensated glass or metal vapourisers may be used in their place, but, though they are cheaper, they are not so easy to manage,[4] so it is best to confine them to the administration of ether. In either case, bellows or bag must be part of the equipment, and this may be obtained locally. Figure 3 shows a diagram of a possible arrangement of a draw over system.

A mask or endotracheal tube may be used for spontaneous respiration, but if this is to be controlled with muscle relaxants an endotracheal tube must be inserted. A trouble free example of a non-rebreathing valve that will function with spontaneous or controlled respiration is the Ambu-E type. This may be copied locally without access to high technology. If there is no valve a finger closing and opening one limb of a Cobb type connector will make controlled ventilation possible (fig 4).

Anaesthetics

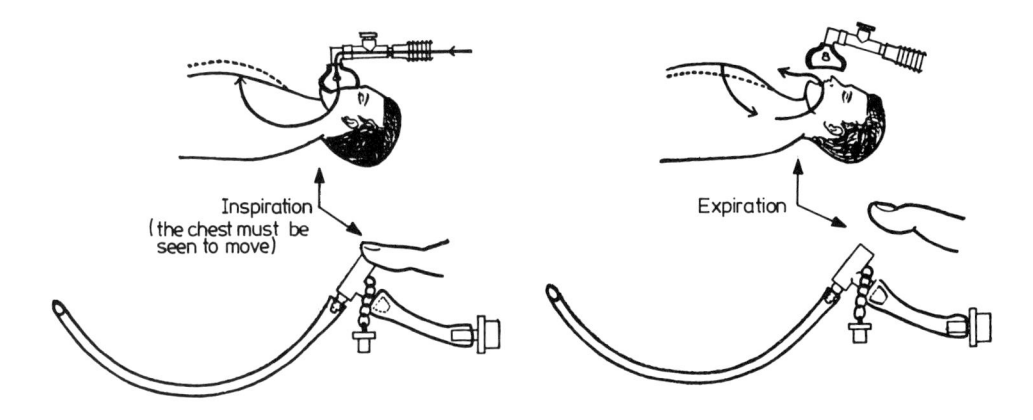

FIG 4—Controlled ventilation when no inflating valve is available, using a mask or endotracheal tube.

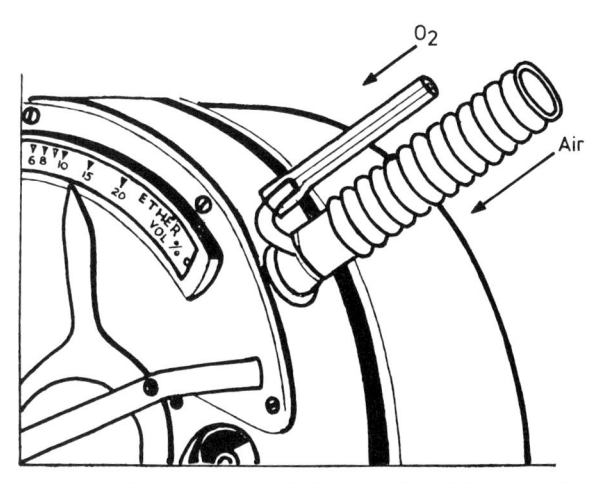

FIG 5—Addition of oxygen to the inspired air, 1-2 l/min, which is sufficient for most patients (shown plugged into the air inlet of an EMO but may be used in the same way with an OMV or Cyprane vapouriser).

It is possible to adapt the bellows for paediatric use by substituting narrow bore tubing from the bellows and connecting it to the gas inlet of an Ayre's T piece. The bellows, which hold 2 litres, can then be operated slowly by hand to produce a nearly continuous flow of 10-12 l/minute.

Oxygen may be added to the inspired air using a simple flow meter. It is connected by a T piece arrangement (fig 5) at the air inlet using about 15 cm of old corrugated tubing, which will ensure that no oxygen is lost up to about 2 l/min flow. Such a flow will give an inhaled concentration of 25-40% depending on the depth of respiration. Oxygen concentrators are now available, but it remains to be seen whether these are going to be practical for general use.

Intubation

The most widely used laryngoscope is the Macintosh, which is curved, the largest blade being preferable, so it can be used without difficulty in normal sized patients while being adequate for those with long necks. For infants and children up to 2 years a straight blade is preferable, and the Seward and Soper blades are good examples. All laryngoscopes are best used with hook on blades.

Disposable plastic endotracheal tubes may be reused safely provided that they are thoroughly cleaned with soap and water and then sterilised in fresh Savlon or Cidex and finally rinsed in sterile water. Red rubber tubes are cheaper and have a longer life. They may be autoclaved or boiled, but it is important to ensure that they are not deformed in any way during the process, or the deformity will become permanent. If the tubes are sealed in brown paper bags before autoclaving they will remain sterile for at least two months.

Ventilators

In place of bellows a ventilator may be incorporated into the system; this is useful for long operations. The simplest is the Radcliffe model which operates the bellows, again as a draw over. If the electricity supply fails the bellows may be detached quickly and worked by hand. A larger model has a direct current motor, which allows it to run off a 12 volt car battery. More versatile but more expensive is the Oxford ventilator.[5] (Prices of equipment mentioned are quoted in table II, where a Boyle's machine is included for comparison.) I should like to emphasise that the equipment described above is adequate for all types of surgery including major thoracic, abdominal, and neurosurgical procedures. It may also be used for respiratory resuscitation by removing the vaporisers. Staff using it should be drilled in the techniques needed for emergency events.

Intravenous anaesthetics

These are usually supplementary to the agents already mentioned rather than alternatives; they should be used only by skilled staff who can readily ventilate the patient. Thiopentone has a good record as long as certain precautions are taken. It should always be given as a 2·5% solution and never stronger. The dose is best limited to 500 mg for an average sized, fit patient and should be scaled down for those who are not fit. The drug should not be used as a sole anaesthetic agent. A range of similar drugs such as methohexitone is available but these have no marked advantages.

Various combinations of narcotics such as morphine 5-10 mg and pethidine 50-100 mg combined with sedative antiemetics such as promethazine 25-50 mg, chlorpromazine 25-50 mg, and lorazepam 1-2 mg may be given by intravenous injection as an adjunct to regional and spinal analgesia. They cannot be used as general anaesthetics. Ketamine (Ketalar), however, may be used as a total anaesthetic, giving complete analgesia and unconsciousness but no muscle relaxation. The dose is 5-10 mg/kg intramuscularly, which lasts about 30 minutes, or 2-4 mg/kg intravenously, which lasts about 10 minutes. The

Anaesthetics

initial dose may be halved for maintenance, or it may be followed by a conventional general anaesthetic used with or without intubation. Intubation must not be attempted with ketamine alone as laryngeal spasm is a real danger; a muscle relaxant should be given in addition. This drug is particularly useful in children for surface operations such as burn grafts, as it is not associated with vomiting and may be used for multiple operations. The disadvantage is that it may produce unpleasant hallucinations, but these may be suppressed with a narcotic or benzodiazepine given preoperatively. Although it is expensive, ketamine is useful and should be stocked for use in selected cases.

Teaching

Anaesthesia may be given simply, but anaesthetic principles need to be scrupulously observed, for it is a thorough understanding of the subject that leads to adaptability and flexibility in practice. In my experience three levels of teaching are needed for those working in the anaesthetic department of a Third World hospital.

(1) Nurses and medical assistants: selected trainees should be taught to become familiar with the apparatus described above. Ideally, these trainees should be taught by the resident anaesthetist, but there are relatively few who have the requisite teaching skills, enthusiasm, and time to undertake this. Hence most trainees will have to be taught in the larger medical centres as near as possible to their own hospital.

(2) Non-specialists: doctors for whom anaesthesia may not be a sole interest or responsibility may be taught on site by the resident anaesthetist.

(3) Specialists in anaesthetics: full time anaesthetic training in recognised centres is needed on a larger scale than is currently available. Specialists need to be taught techniques that are appropriate to the countries in which they work, and unfortunately, at present, few centres give this sort of training, with the result that most trainees get the idea that without a Boyle's or Heidbrink machine nothing can be done.

In my view, promoting and encouraging appropriate anaesthetic training programmes is essential. (A detailed teaching manual called *Primary anaesthesia* will be published by the World Health Organisation before the end of 1984, which will be suitable for use in training both doctors and auxiliaries.) By this means, and using the simple equipment described above, any form of surgery may be undertaken and a standard of anaesthesia maintained that is equally as good as that in Western countries.

References

[1] Roberts JG, Prys-Roberts C, Moore MA, Frazer ANI. Cardiopulmonary function during ether/air relaxant anaesthesia. A comparison with nitrous oxide/oxygen anaesthesia. *Anaesthesia* 1974;**29**:4-16.
[2] Prior FN. Trichloroethylene in air with muscle relaxants. *Anaesthesia* 1972;**27**:66-75.
[3] Houghton IT. The Triservice anaesthetic apparatus. *Anaesthesia* 1981;**36**:1094-108, 1112-27.
[4] Boulton TB, Cole PR. Anaesthesia in difficult situations. *Anaesthesia* 1966;**21**:268, 379, 513 and 1967;**22**:101, 435.
[5] Sugg BR, Prys-Roberts C. The Penlon Oxford ventilator. A new ventilator for adult or paediatric use. *Anaesthesia* 1976;**31**:1234-44.

Recommended reading

Farman J. *Anaesthesia and the EMO system.* Kent: English Universities Press, 1973.
Atkinson RS, Rushman GB, Lee JA. *Synopsis of anaesthesia.* Bristol: Wright, 1982.
Prior FN. *A manual of anaesthesia for the small hospital.* 2nd ed. New Delhi: Voluntary Health Association of India, 1977.
Macintosh RR, Ostlere M. *Local analgesia—head and neck.* Edinburgh: Livingstone, 1955.
Macintosh RR, Bryce-Smith R. *Local analgesia—abdominal surgery.* Edinburgh: Livingstone, 1953.
Lee JA, Atkinson RS. *Lumbar puncture and spinal analgesia.* London: Longman, 1978.
Eriksson E. *Illustrated handbook of local anaesthesia.* Denmark: Munksgaard, 1979.
Lee JA, Bryce-Smith R. *Practical regional analgesia.* Amsterdam: Excerpta Medica, Elsevier, 1976.

Manufacturers in the United Kingdom (who also give information on overseas agents).

EMO/OMV/Oxford ventilator, laryngoscopes, and endotracheal tubes. Penlon Ltd, Abingdon, Bucks OX14 3PH.
Radcliffe ventilator. H G East & Co Ltd, Sandy Lane W, Littlemore, Oxford OX4 5JT.
Cyprane vapourisers. Cyprane, New Devonshire House, Scott Street, Keighley, Bucks BD21 2NN.

EPIDEMIOLOGY AND RESEARCH AT LOW COST

PETER COX

At first sight it would seem that both research and epidemiology are high technology, high cost activities carried out by highly qualified specialists with nothing else to do except punch buttons on computers or organise well trained scientists working in well equipped laboratories. This is not so, for good epidemiological data should be the basis for all health planning from national to district level, and the more scanty the resources the more accurate the decisions must be. The data needed by the district medical officer for day to day decisions in planning the number of beds in a health centre or determining the size of a new hospital are also the bricks and mortar of the nation's statistics. The morbidity figures reported in the dispensaries make up the country's health statistics. Hence inaccurate, deficient, or out of date figures at district level may lead to poor planning and a distorted picture of the overall health problems of the country.

This article aims at encouraging those at the periphery of the health network to improve their methods of collecting data and embark on the vital basic research that only they can do. These tasks are not optional extras: they should be priorities in the schedule of every district medical officer.

Establishing a baseline

One of the great difficulties in working in developing countries, especially as a newcomer to a remote district, is the lack of a baseline. What is normal? Values may vary among ethnic groups, among neighbouring districts, or even among villages as little as 30 or 40 miles apart. In one district in which I worked the serum protein concentrations showed a wide variation among four centres of population, and all these concentrations were higher than those in adjoining districts and tribes.[1] Disease prevalence may vary with altitude and climate and be profoundly influenced by the local customs and way of life. This was so noticeable in one district that it was virtually possible to predict the patient's home area from his symptoms.[2] Attendances may vary from month to month according to the season and are often dictated far more by social, geographic, and agricultural factors than purely medical ones. The district medical officer must find and record these idiosyncrasies and interpret the regional statistics against this background, for without this interpretation a misleading picture may be drawn. For example, in one tribe the incidence of tapeworm in men was about four times that in the women. Many years elapsed before we found that the people believed that possession of a tapeworm increased the chances of pregnancy. The picture was spurious for the actual incidence was the same, but the women did not come for treatment.

The pattern of disease

It is vital to work out an accurate pattern of disease for the district as a whole, and to be aware of the variations present in each part of the district. The first stage may be to get a broad distribution of the conditions seen in the outpatient department, which will probably be a mixture of diseases such as measles or malaria and symptoms such as headache and abdominal discomfort from splenomegaly. Staff should be encouraged to record symptoms accurately rather than make wild guesses at a diagnosis, as did one ungraded dresser in a remote dispensary, who diagnosed all his headaches as cancer of the brain. Fortunately, the district medical officer spotted the error before the figures reached the World Health Organisation in Geneva. The second stage is to examine these symptoms or syndromes by measuring them, reaching a firm diagnosis, if possible, and feeding back the information to the primary health care worker.

Attendances and morbidity figures may be represented graphically on a chart, which is the most effective way to show fluctuations or rising and falling trends. Attendances should be charted monthly as well as annually, to pick out seasonal variations due to migration, climate, or agricultural activity, along with the rising or falling use of each medical unit. It is particularly useful to have a graph of the rainfall to compare with the changing incidence of conditions such as malaria and gastroenteritis, for it may be possible to predict seasonal epidemics and take appropriate action. Finally, a large scale map should be drawn to show the whole district on one sheet. Mark each health delivery point and draw a five mile circle round it to get an idea of the health coverage and distance people have to travel for aid. Mark every place visited regularly by mobile health units or community workers. Flags or pins may be used to indicate specific problems and by this means disease foci may be located—for example, cases of brucellosis round an infected milk herd.

The tally survey

The tally survey is a simple method of collecting data in a given area, using existing health care staff to collect additional information in the course of their routine work. The method is flexible and may be applied to a variety of problems, from recording attendances at the outpatient department to determining infant mortality. It is also useful in supplementing the statutory returns and giving some body of fact to an impression or hunch about the occurrence of a particular disorder. The specific rules vary with each survey and they must be defined clearly and in great detail so that the same question is asked by each worker and their measurements are made in the same way. Directions should be printed on each tally sheet, and if possible

Epidemiology and research at low cost

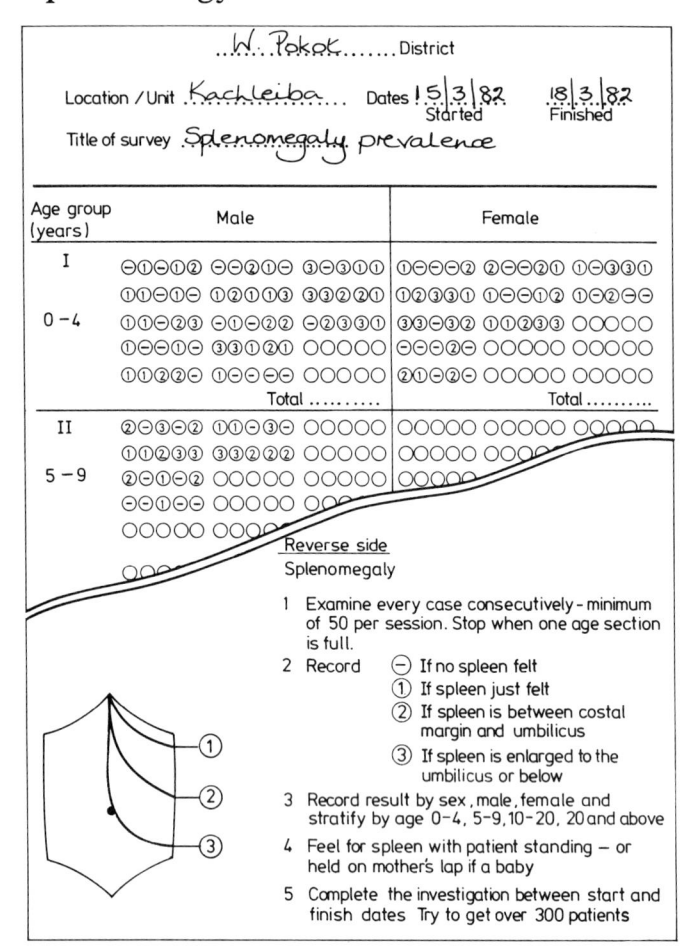

FIG 1—Tally survey.

The advantages of the tally survey are that we get a large volume of information on each fact, the survey may be repeated at any time, and the staff get into the habit of routinely observing and recording background data. The disadvantage is that the sample is inevitably biased by recording only attenders, though this is offset by the large numbers of healthy people attending mobile clinics and if home visitors of any category are used. Indeed, for certain facts, such as the prevalence of blindness or disability from polio, only the use of home visitors will give any indication of the true figures as people thus affected tend not to leave their homes.

Estimation of population

The major difficulty in establishing accurate health statistics for a district or area lies in enumerating the total population. The official census may be out of date, and in a remote area, almost certainly an underestimate. One useful method of overcoming this is to ask any visitor coming to the district by air to take photographs with a handheld camera of a specific area of interest (fig 2). The farmsteads and houses may easily be counted, and a quick check on the ground will give the average number of occupants for each house.

Chiefs, elders, and administrative officers are likely to be good sources of local knowledge and will probably be able to list the main families in an area. Schoolchildren may also be able to give the numbers in their households and identify the blind and paralysed people confined to the houses.

the district medical officer or a senior deputy should explain them to each person doing the recording. An example of a tally sheet used to assess the prevalence of splenomegaly is shown in fig 1. The workers must appreciate that they must record negative as well as positive results, and the district medical officer must ensure that they understand what they are doing and why.[3] Some short rationale for the investigation may also be printed on the sheet—for example, "The common causes of splenomegaly in our district are malaria, brucellosis, and kala azar. We want to find out how many people have large spleens so that we can find the proper diagnosis and arrange for the proper treatment of each patient."

Other investigations may be carried out by modifying the stratification of the age groups, by contrasting school against village children or one ethnic group against another. Simple background data on such things as the prevalence of goitre, dental caries, blindness, or disability from poliomyelitis may easily be obtained by following this method. More uncommon conditions, in which a rate is not required, may be estimated by recording every positive case for a month and merely matching this against the total monthly attendance. In establishing the infant mortality rate every woman is asked "How many children have you delivered?" and "How many of those children are alive?" The first answer is recorded on the left side and the second in the equivalent position on the right. A similar recording may be used for the stillbirth or abortion rate.

It is useful to use every medical unit in the district to collect data, and in certain simple investigations using school teachers, social workers, nutritionists, and family planning workers will achieve a wide coverage. This would be particularly useful in estimating the number of attendances at a health unit compared with the distance of the residence from it, when the stratifications would show the distance from the health unit and the number of visits would be recorded in each space.

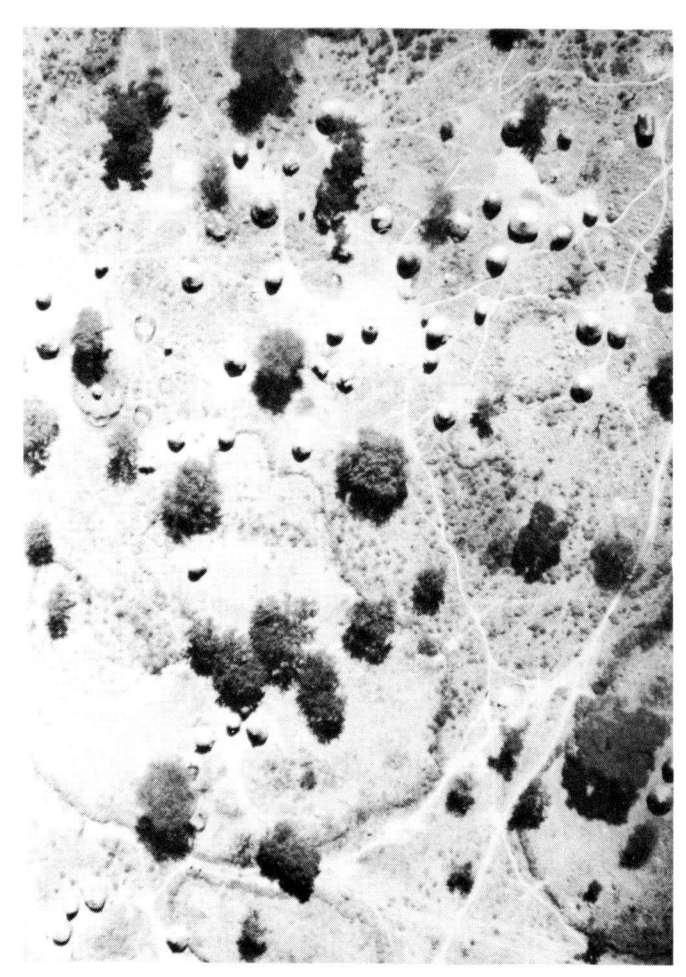

FIG 2—In remote areas estimates of population may be aided by taking aerial photographs and counting the number of houses.

Research

Collection of basic data inevitably uncovers problems and eventually leads to simple research. Much tremendously useful work may be done by the district medical officer, either in collaboration with a central laboratory or by using existing laboratory facilities and simple tests. Most of these tests would be carried out routinely for diagnostic purposes in any case, but as results accumulate and records are brought together valuable information is found and a general picture begins to emerge. For instance, the splenomegaly that has now been proved to exist and to be a major problem as a result of the tally survey may be investigated further. Perhaps three quarters of all children under 5 have large spleens and half of the adults as well. The routine tests have shown that malaria, kala azar, and brucellosis exist, although the prevalence of each is not known. The district medical officer may make an attempt to solve this problem by collating the clinical tests and making sure that a simple protocol is adhered to in every case.

For instance, a directive is issued to all staff interviewing and treating patients:

"Please refer all patients with grade 2 or 3 spleens to the district medical officer or take a coagulated and non-coagulated blood sample from each case and send to the laboratory."

The laboratory will carry out the following tests on every sample: haemoglobin, white cell count, thin and thick blood slide, formol gel, brucella rapid slide test. Spleen punctures or marrow biopsy may be carried out in some cases as a second stage and if possible the results of treatment collated with the results.

The results are then sufficient for a firm report to be sent to the ministry of health and a collaborative survey to be undertaken with the vets or vector borne diseases units and above all for a rational scheme of treatment to be carried out by local staff.

The classic example of the way in which simple mapping of the occurrence of a condition may lead to the recognition of a new disease must surely be the investigation of African lymphoma by Dennis Burkitt. He observed the correlation between the number of cases and the altitude, and then the distribution of the *Anopheles* mosquito and malaria. Further research linked the tumour with the Epstein-Barr virus and unravelled the immunological relation with malaria, while he and other workers were able to carry out work on the histological appearance of the tumour and methods of treatment.[5][6]

The key to low cost and low technology research is to pick subjects that depend on the observation or occurrence in a specific locality, backed up by very simple tests. It is particularly important to link this type of research to local knowledge. Two examples might be cited. Firstly, the apparently unique occurrence of procidentia in young women of low parity. This was tackled by sending a simple questionnaire to about 50 neighbouring hospitals, asking about female circumcision, the ethnic population served, and whether prolapse of the uterus occurred. It seemed, when all this information was returned, that the problem was unique to the district and was due to the custom of the local midwives to press hard on the fundus in early labour.[7] The second problem was the occurrence of a severe arthritis, in one area, affecting hip, knee, and spine. This was solved by carrying out a survey using the rose bengal slide agglutination test for brucellosis, when about 38% of the tested cases were found to be positive each year. This investigation was repeated in other areas, where constant figures were again obtained.[7]

Merely keeping a register of certain conditions will lead to valuable information being recorded. Certainly every hospital should have a cancer register, and, while it might prove impossible for a district medical officer to carry out complete tests on thyroid function, all known cases of goitre may be recorded and mapped so that a future research worker may have months of time saved.

In summary, collect, record, and report the facts and findings from your district—what may be familiar and commonplace to you may be rare and interesting to someone else. Carry out your own bits of research as far as you can go, for it is very likely that you may supply the very information that the high technology scientist lacks.

The Makerere team, in Uganda, in the 1960s enlisted the cooperation of all the peripheral hospitals in the investigation of the tropical splenomegaly syndrome; surely this is how research should be done with low cost intermediate technology paving the way, or working in conjunction with the university team.

References

[1] Cox PSV. The disease pattern of the karapokot. London: London University, 1972. (MD thesis.)
[2] Cox PSV. Geographical variation of disease within a single district. *East Afr Med J* 1973;**50**:712-9.
[3] Maar EWJ, Chaudhury RR, Ekue JMK, Franata F, Walker AN. Management of clinical trials in developing countries. *J Int Med Res* 1983;**11**:1-5.
[5] Burkitt D. Determining the climatic limitations of a children's cancer common in Africa. *Br Med J* 1962;**ii**:1019-23.
[6] Burkitt D, Wright D. Geographical and tribal distribution of the African lymphoma in Uganda. *Br Med J* 1966;**i**:569-73.
[7] Cox PSV, Webster D. Genital prolapse. *East Afr Med J* 1975;**52**:694-9.
[8] Cox PSV. Brucellosis—a survey in South Karamoja. *East Afr Med J* 1966;**43**:43-50.

PRIORITIES FOR HOSPITAL CLEANING, DISINFECTION, STERILISATION, AND CONTROL OF INFECTION

ROSEMARY SIMPSON

The continuing high prevalence of infectious diseases in developing countries—in contrast to the dramatic decline of such diseases in the West—has been attributed to many factors, among which poor sanitation and hygiene, inadequate medical services, and malnutrition are foremost. In this article I consider what measures may be taken in a district hospital in the Third World, to help in controlling infection and achieving a reasonable standard of hygiene. In developing countries policies for the treatment and control of infectious disease need to be geared to the specific needs of the community and take into account the fact that many hospitals have no electricity, an inadequate water supply, and no reliable sewage facilities. Such circumstances necessitate a simplified and more fundamental approach that is both economically viable and effective. Although direct comparison with standards feasible in the West may not always be appropriate, it may be beneficial in stimulating a re-examination of conventional and possibly wasteful practices.

Limited resources and adverse geographical factors are important considerations in formulating public health policies, but effective health measures also call for understanding the local cultural practices and religious beliefs. Various approaches have been made—for example, that put forward by the Environmental Health Division of the Royal Army Medical Training Group, Keogh Barracks, Ash Vale, Aldershot, Hants. Other organisations that provide advice and training schemes on various aspects of public health are listed at the end of this article.

Water supply

A safe, clean water supply is essential. A piped supply is preferable, but water from a field deep well or standing tank collecting rainwater is adequate. The first step is purification, which entails removing suspended organic matter by filtering the water through mechanical pressure filters—for example, the Voges filter—or by slow sedimentation. For some purposes this may be all that is required, but water for drinking requires further measures to destroy contaminating micro-organisms. This may be done by fixed dose chlorination (minimum residual chlorine level 2 ppm), preferably using a chlorinator (sodium thiosulphate may then be added to improve the taste), or by adding water purification tablets.

Sterile bottled water may be prepared in the hospital provided that high standards are maintained in distillation and sterilisation. An autoclave specifically designed to take bottled fluids is necessary, and this must be in good working order. Alternatively, sterile bottled water may be bought, but it is likely to be expensive. Irrespective of the source, care must be taken in the storage of all sterile fluids and the containers must be critically examined regularly; if there is any evidence of defective sealing or contamination of the fluids they must not be used. Once the container has been opened the contents should be used straight away or rejected. Boiled water is not sterile and should not be used to make up solutions for intravenous use. Boiling does, however, reduce the bacterial and viral load to a safe level for drinking and for making up oral rehydration fluid and powdered infant feed.

Waste disposal and sewage

Effective disposal of human excreta and hospital refuse is vital to combat the spread of disease carried by flies and rats. The best way to dispose of hospital waste is to burn it in an incinerator in the hospital grounds or a safe site elsewhere. Incinerators may be made from empty metal drums or sheets of corrugated iron (figure). Waste for incineration should be taken to a designated area and stored in lidded bins until burnt. A piped sewage system to either a mains sewer or a septic tank is the best way to dispose of human excreta, but such a system is practicable only if the water supply is ample and uninterrupted. An alternative method is to dig deep trench latrines (which should be covered to exclude flies) or ventilated pit latrines and improvised urinals with soakage pits. Both hospital staff and patients need to be taught that many diseases, especially gastrointestinal disorders, may be spread by the faecal/oral route, and advice on basic hygiene must be an integral part of any community health education programme. In the hospital ward urinals and bedpans should be removed from the patient immediately after use and the contents disposed of in a designated area. Pans should then be thoroughly cleaned and disinfected in a separate area well away from food—preferably with hot water (80°C) or, alternatively, by immersion in a disinfectant. Laboratory waste such as discarded cultures and specimens should be rendered safe to handle by autoclaving before transporting in sealed containers to a designated site for incineration.

Sterilisation of instruments and dressings

Sterilisation by heat is the method of choice in the hospital. Unwrapped metal or glass instruments may be processed either by moist heat in a simple downward displacement autoclave

Priorities for hospital cleaning and control of infection

or by dry heat in a hot air oven. Porous loads such as dressings must only be processed in the more complex high vacuum cycle autoclaves. Selection of the most up to date machines is not always wise (and may be expensive), for they may break down if the steam supply is poor or intermittent and are difficult to repair. Provided that the standard conditions of temperatures and time recommended by the Medical Research Council are met and the recommended procedures carried out,[1][2] a simple machine design is quite adequate. One such example is the multipurpose compact autoclave (manufactured by Thackray), which is suitable for sterilising wrapped and unwrapped instruments, dressings and other porous articles, and bottled fluids. The machine is manually operated and runs off either a direct steam supply or clean cold water that is heated up by electricity.

Autoclaves that operate on a fully automatic cycle reduce operator errors but need trained staff to check that the machine achieves the necessary cycle characteristics. Simple autoclaves built on similar lines to a pressure cooker and heated by wood or electricity may be used to sterilise unwrapped instruments and utensils and are more effective than simply putting them in boiling water. Unwrapped instruments should be used immediately after sterilisation. If allowed to dry and then stored in clean conditions the instruments may get recontaminated and will need to be sterilised again before use. Wrapped sterile instruments, disposable syringes, needles, and fine catheters should be stored carefully in lidded boxes in a dry site away from direct sunlight, direct heat, and vermin. The expense and restricted availability of prepacked items will preclude their use in many hospitals, so it is advisable to buy items that are made of material that may be recycled.

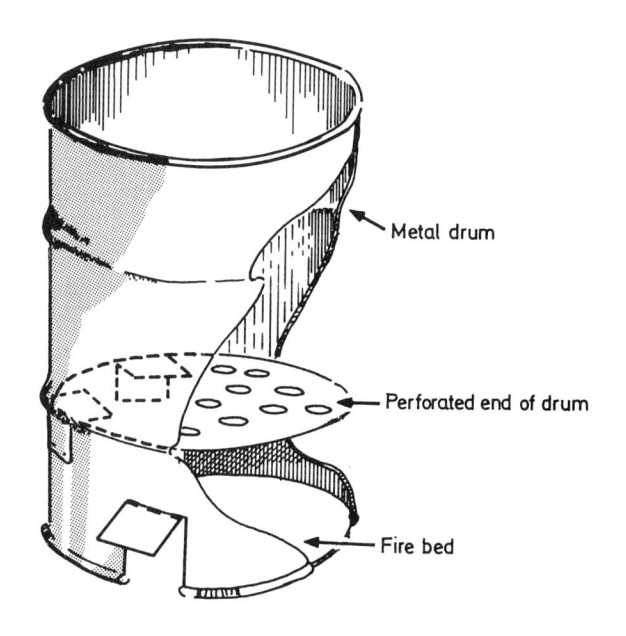

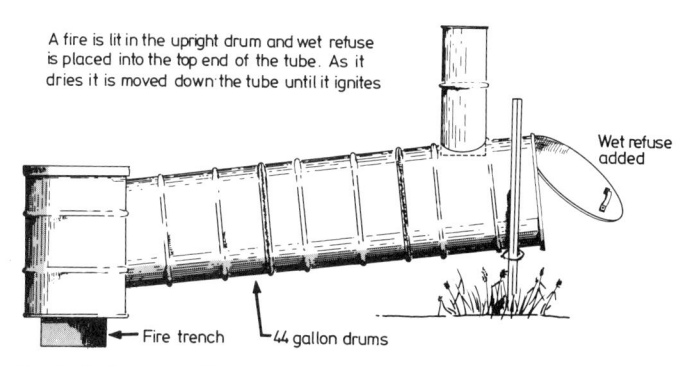

Simple incinerators. (Drawing based on illustrations in *Sketches of Field Hygiene Appliances*, 1st Preventive Medicine Company, Ingleb.)

Cleaning the hospital

Cleaning walls and other flat surfaces is easier if the surfaces are reasonably smooth, so the junction between walls and floors should be covered and crevices sealed. Dusting or sweeping floors with brushes impregnated with water or oil or used tea leaves helps discourage dust from rising up. Floors should be kept socially clean by the most appropriate method for the type of surface. For washing floors and other surfaces a detergent and soap solution is sufficient. Cotton floor mops should be washed after use and dried thoroughly in direct sunlight with the head uppermost before being put away. Walls, floors, and furniture need to be disinfected only if contaminated with potentially infected material, for example, faeces, urine, or blood. Lavatories should be thoroughly cleaned and disinfected twice a day, or more frequently as necessary.

Throughout the hospital care needs to be taken to ensure that the ventilation is adequate. Movement of insects through open windows may be reduced by putting up mesh screening.

Care in the kitchen

Kitchen staff need to be trained to maintain high standards of hygiene to prevent outbreaks of food poisoning and the transmission of other gastrointestinal infections. Handwashing before and after preparing food is essential, and plenty of readily accessible hand wash basins need to be provided. Cooked and uncooked food should be handled separately and stored in separate, covered containers. Refrigeration facilities are important and must be well maintained. All work surfaces should be easy to clean.

Staff should be aware of the length of cooking time required to destroy microbes in meat and poultry, and the possibility of there being carriers of enteric pathogens not only among catering staff but also throughout the hospital. Food prepared for individual patients by their relatives is another possible source of contaminated food entering the hospital.

Laundry

Separate laundry facilities with reliable machines to do really hot washes are the optimum. Simple jacketed machines using steam heated by a wood fire may be just as effective as Western style machines. If no machines are available washing by hand using hot water followed by drying in direct sunshine is adequate because ultraviolet rays have an appreciable disinfectant action. Soaking laundry in large containers of disinfectant is not a good way to clean it. Soiled articles should be placed in sealed bags or covered containers in a designated area and washed properly as soon as possible.

Disinfection

Every hospital needs a disinfectant policy, and staff should be taught how to use disinfectants at the recommended concentration following the manufacturer's instructions. I suggest that the following types of disinfectant should be stocked:

(1) General purpose clear soluble phenols such as Lysol or Clearsol to be used in conditions where organic soiling is high—for example, faecally contaminated sites.

(2) Hypochlorites such as Chloros and Domestos are rapidly acting inexpensive disinfectants that are suitable for the disinfection of surfaces contaminated by blood and for wiping down surfaces on which food is prepared.

(3) Two per cent buffered glutaraldehydes are expensive but a good way to decontaminate heat labile equipment such as transducers or fibreoptic endoscopes. (Their relative toxicity and expense preclude their use as general purpose disinfectants.)

(4) Skin disinfectants, such as Hibitane and Betadine, may be

Priorities for hospital cleaning and control of infection

used as detergent based emulsions with water or as alcohol preparations.

Hospital staff need to get into the habit of regular handwashing, but this is possible only if there are enough wash basins throughout the hospital, and ideally these should have a continuous supply of soap and clean disposable towels. Alcoholic disinfectant preparations, such as Hibisol, are more effective than their aqueous counterparts and may be used as well as basic soap and water for procedures that require a high standard of cleanliness. Many procedures are best carried out with sterile gloves, but if supplies are restricted great emphasis must be placed on scrupulous hand disinfection.

Additional measures

Control of antibiotic prescription by an agreed hospital policy is an important part of any policy to control hospital infection. Indiscriminate use of antibiotics increases the incidence of infection with resistant bacteria. If possible, arrangements should be made to isolate patients with serious and contagious infections and to carry out barrier nursing if necessary. Reasonable standards of health care can be maintained only through the cooperation of all the hospital staff. Greater awareness of the essential facts about the spread of disease and how to carry out the measures described above should ensure that a reasonable standard of hygiene is maintained in the hospital.

I am grateful to the following colleagues in the preparation of this article: Professor W A Gillespie, department of microbiology, Bristol Royal Infirmary; Major B Hart, Environmental Health Division, RAMC Training Group; Mr W J Jones, consultant engineer for Crown Agents for Overseas Governments and Administrations; Miss Annette Viant, nursing officer infection control, Bristol Royal Infirmary; and Miss Elizabeth Jenner, nursing officer, Whittington Hospital.

References

[1] Working party on Pressure-steam Sterilisers. *Sterilisation by steam under increased pressure.* London: Medical Research Council, 1959.
[2] Medical Research Council. Memorandum. London: MRC, 1962. (MRC Memorandum No 41.)

Organisations that give advice on public health measures

(1) Environmental Health Division, Royal Army Medical Training Group, Keogh Barracks, Ash Vale, Nr Aldershot, Hants.
(2) Hospital Estate Management and Engineering Centre, Eastwood Park, Falfield, Gloucestershire GL12 8DA. (Provides regular training courses abroad for engineers and other hospital staff.)
(3) Infection Control Nurses Association, secretary Miss G Weymont, senior nurse, infection control, Royal United Hospital, Bath. (Provides advice, training schemes, and teaching aids for nurses in infection control.)
(4) Central Sterilising Club, honorary secretary Dr R A Simpson, Department of Microbiology, Bristol Royal Infirmary, Bristol BS2 8HW. (A multi-professional society offering advice on all aspects of disinfection, sterilisation, and infection control in the hospital.)
(5) Division of Hospital Infection, director Professor E M Cooke, Central Public Health Laboratory, Colindale Avenue, London NW9 5HT.
(6) Hospital Infection Research Laboratory, director Professor G A J Ayliffe, Dudley Road, Birmingham B18 7QH.

Recommended reading

Aspects of Infection Control, a series of free booklets available from Pharmaceutical Division, Imperial Chemical Industries plc, Alderley Park, Cheshire. Useful titles in the series are:
Ojajarui J. *Hands as vectors of disease.*
Nyström MD. *The disinfection of objects and inanimate surfaces in hospitals.*
Alder VG. *Central sterile supply and medical equipment decontamination centres.*
Lowbury EJL, Ayliffe GAJ, Geddes AM, Williams JD, eds. *Control of hospital infection. A practical handbook.* 2nd ed. London: Chapman and Hall, 1981.
Ayliffe GAJ, Collins BJ, Taylor LJ. *Hospital acquired infection, principles and prevention.* Bristol: John Wright, 1982.
Maur IM. *Hospital hygiene.* 2nd ed. London: Arnold, 1978.
Bennett JV, Brachman PS, eds. *Hospital infections.* Boston: Little Brown, 1979.
Ayliffe GAJ, ed. *The Journal of Hospital Infection.* Academic Press in association with the Hospital Infection Society.

LABORATORY EQUIPMENT—WHERE ARE THE TOOLS TO DO THE WORK?

MONICA CHEESBROUGH

The call for appropriate technology in medical laboratory sciences, especially for equipment, is becoming widespread and urgent. In developed countries new technology has led to a proliferation of complex tools and a tendency to overinvestigate patients. Such tools have been introduced more in response to demand than need, with the tacit help of manufacturers. For many health authorities this costly new technology is becoming difficult to sustain.

In the Third World it is a question not of financial cuts threatening existing services but of how to establish a service at all when the tools do not exist or, if they are available, are often too expensive. It is a disturbing fact that (with few exceptions) none of the commercial manufacturers' profits have been used to research appropriate tools for use in developing countries.

Which investigations?

Before considering which tools are necessary in a district hospital laboratory in a developing country it is helpful to look at the range of tests that are currently undertaken in these laboratories (table I). Not all the tests listed will be required in every district hospital laboratory, and it may be necessary to include others. Tests should always be selected according to local health needs, cost effectiveness, training and experience of laboratory staff, reagents and equipment needed, and whether a reliable referral system is available. Owing to high cost, lack of facilities, and inexperienced staff, many district laboratories find it difficult or impossible to estimate serum electrolyte concentrations or to carry out culture and sensitivity tests.

It is important to have close links with a regional laboratory to ensure the reliability of the peripheral service and to allow more complex biochemical and serological tests to be carried out. It may also be possible to refer microbiological specimens—for example, sputum for the culture of *Mycobacterium tuberculosis*, urogenital swabs for *Neisseria gonorrhoeae*, and throat swabs for group A *Streptococcus*. All specimens must be collected and preserved correctly.[1] A referral system usually operates between the provincial or central laboratory and the peripheral laboratories for the examination of smears for malignant cells, histological examination of biopsy specimens, and reporting of bone marrow aspirates.

Table II shows the range of equipment needed to perform the investigations listed in table I. Guidelines for the specifications of these items of equipment may be found in a document published by the World Health Organisation.[2] For descriptions and ordering information about most of the equipment in this list, readers are referred to chapters two, three, and five in volume 1 of a *Medical Laboratory Manual for Tropical Countries*.[1]

The equipment listed in table II is neither extensive nor complex, yet few peripheral laboratories have these basic resources—a fact which underlies a recent statement from the World Health Organisation that "... every aspect of the supply and operation of health care laboratory equipment in developing countries is seriously deficient ... a rigorous programme of design, supply, maintenance, and repair must be established in all countries."[3]

Equipment must be designed for its environment

An instrument that has been designed to operate in a laboratory in a developed country by trained scientists with regular servicing by skilled engineers is destined for a short and difficult life in the district laboratory of a developing country. Even if it survives the journey, the circuit shorting, mould growing and heat of the wet season, the dust of the dry season, and the intermittent electrical supplies, its end will surely come when a vital part cannot be obtained, or the laboratory assistant or local car mechanic takes a look inside and attempts to repair it without recourse to a maintenance or service manual. Equipment for use in a developing country peripheral laboratory must meet certain criteria. It must:

(1) Be rugged, and able to operate reliably under extremes of heat, humidity, and drought.

(2) Be fitted with a voltage stabiliser if indicated.

(3) Be designed for easy use by those with limited technical training and experience.

(4) Come ready supplied with essential spare parts and a clearly written and illustrated maintenance and service manual.

Basic care and preventive maintenance of laboratory equipment should be included in the syllabuses of all laboratory workers, and every developing country should establish a centre for servicing equipment and evaluating the suitability of new equipment. These and other aspects of equipment design and care have been discussed at length.[3]

Battery or mains operated equipment

Many district hospitals in developing countries are without 24 hour mains electricity and are served only by a generator. This may operate only when the main hospital autoclave is used, when major surgery is performed, and for a few hours each evening to light the wards when darkness falls. (Kerosene lamps take over when the generator "sleeps.") Even if the hospital does have mains electricity, electrical supplies are often intermittent and of irregular voltage. Thus it is necessary to find alternative power supplies and adapt and redesign equipment to operate from these. Solar powered cells are expensive, so a 12 volt lead acid storage battery, rechargeable from the mains when operating, or possibly from a windmill, is the power pack of choice.

Laboratory equipment—where are the tools to do the work?

TABLE I—*Laboratory tests performed in district hospitals in developing countries**

Investigation	Usual method	Investigation	Usual method
Blood		*Skin*	
Haemoglobin concentration	Colorimetric	Smears for *Mycobacterium leprae*	Ziehl-Neelsen
Total white cell count	Counting chamber	Snips for *Onchocerca volvulus*	Saline preparation
Differential white cell count and red cell morphology	Examination of stained thin film	Scrapings for fungi	Potassium hydroxide preparation
Platelet count	Counting chamber	*Sputum*	
Reticulocyte count	Examination of stained preparation	Smear for tubercle bacilli	Ziehl-Neelsen
Packed cell volume	Centrifuge	Detection of eosinophils	Eosin preparation
Mean cell haemoglobin concentration	Calculation from haemoglobin concentration and packed cell volume	*Paragonimus* eggs	Saline preparation
Erythrocyte sedimentation rate	Westergren	*Exudate and discharges*	
Bleeding time	Filter paper method	Pus for gonococci	Gram smear
Clotting time	Lee and White tube method	Vaginal discharge for *Trichomonas* and *Candida*	Saline preparation, Gram smear if parasites and yeasts are not detected
Blood grouping	Slide (tile) and tube methods	Ulcer exudate for donovanosis	Giemsa smear for Leishman-Donovan bodies
Compatibility testing	Room temperature saline, antihuman globulin (if available) or albumin at 37°C	Chancre fluid for syphilis	Dark field for spirochaetes
		Mucopus from mycetoma or eumycetoma (granules)	Potassium hydroxide preparation
Antibody testing:			
To investigate syphilis	Rapid plasma reagin (RPR) card test or Venereal Diseases Reference Laboratory (VDRL)	*Urine*	
To investigate enteric fever	Slide and tube agglutination	Cells, casts, bacteria, crystals	Direct microscopy (Gram of sediment if pus cells present)
To investigate brucellosis	Slide and tube agglutination	Protein	Reagent strip test or sulphosalicylic acid test
Blood glucose concentration	Colorimetric		
Blood urea concentration	Colorimetric	Glucose	Reagent strip test or Benedict's test
Serum bilirubin concentration	Colorimetric	Ketones	Reagent strip or tablet test or nitroprusside test
Total protein concentration	Colorimetric	Bilirubin	Fouchet's test
Malaria parasites	Field's stained thick smear, Giemsa stained thin smear, buffy coat stained smear	Urobilinogen	Ehrlich's tube test
		Haemoglobin	Reagent strip test
Trypanosomes	Field's stained thick smear, direct microscopy of plasma in microhaematocrit	Pregnancy test	Slide test to detect human chorionic gonadotrophin (HCG), tube test to semiquantify HCG
Microfilariae	Lysed blood preparation, direct microscopy of plasma in microhaematocrit, haematoxylin and eosin smear	*Schistosoma haematobium*	Direct microscopy for eggs and red cells, or membrane filtration, Schisto-kit, also a test for protein
Borreliae	Field's stained thick smear	*Faeces*	
Screening test for kala-azar	Formol gel test	Parasites	Direct microscopy for amoebae, cysts, larvae, and eggs, using saline, eosin, and iodine. Concentration technique for eggs, especially of schistosomes
Sickle cell test	Sodium metabisulphite slide test, sodium dithionite tube test, Romanowsky stained blood film		
Cerebrospinal fluid		Occult blood	Peroheme-40 (British Drug Houses (BDH) test)
Cell count	Counting chamber	*Other*	
Cell differential	Romanowsky stained smear	Lactase deficiency	Benedict's test or Clinitest to detect sugar (lactose). Strip test to detect low pH
Pyogenic bacteria	Gram smear		
Tubercle bacilli	Ziehl-Neelsen smear		
Protein	Sulphosalicylic acid test		
Globulin screen	Pandy's phenol test		
Glucose estimation	Colorimetric		
Trypanosomes and Mott cells	Direct microscopy and Giemsa smear		

* Not all the tests listed will be required in every district hospital laboratory, and it may also be necessary to include others.

TABLE II—*Equipment required for district laboratories in developing countries*

Major equipment	Additional equipment	
Microscope	Bunsen burner or spirit lamp	Slides and coverglasses
Centrifuge	Hot plate	Syringes, needles, blood lancets
Heat block or water bath	Insulated container	Forceps
Haemoglobin meter or colorimeter (or both)	Differential cell counter	Tourniquet
Water filter	Hand tally counter	Blood taking sets
Water still	Counting chambers	Dressings
Steriliser	Interval timer	Cleaning materials
Refrigerator	Dispensing and pipetting devices	Markers
Balance	Racks and trays	Thermometer
	Staining equipment	Glass and plastic ware to collect, test, and disinfect specimens and to prepare and store stains and reagents
	pH meter or narrow range pH papers	

At present the range of laboratory equipment that runs off a battery is limited and usually expensive, but there is a new company—Primary Health Equipment Ltd—that has been formed recently to design and produce inexpensive laboratory equipment, especially battery operated equipment, for use in peripheral laboratories in developing countries.

Details of essential equipment

MICROSCOPE

The microscope is the most important tool in the laboratory, but although the range is vast, there is at present no instrument that is ideally suited for use in a district laboratory in a developing country. Such a microscope should be rugged, tropicalised, and able to be serviced by the user. An instrument equipped with a mirror and battery operated lamp is required for hospitals without mains electricity. Daylight is not sufficient for use with the oil immersion objective, especially when the microscope is binocular. A low priced, ruggedly built range of microscopes is the Zenith range, available from Primary Health Equipment Ltd. The binocular quadruple nosepiece model is shown in figure 1. It is equipped with a mechanical stage, condenser and iris, and range of optics to give magnifications up to × 1350. It costs £247 complete with case and three objectives. Available accessories include a dark ground condenser (price £19), a lamp unit for mains electricity supply, a × 60 oil immersion lens, and other optics. Monocular instruments are also available from £150, complete with optics, mechanical stage, mirror, and case.

For those who require a compact portable microscope the small in focus McArthur microscope is available from McArthur Microscopes Ltd. It costs £494 and comes complete with optics. A range of accessories is available.

CENTRIFUGE

This is required to separate whole blood to obtain serum for cross matching, serological tests, and biochemical tests and to obtain sediments of cerebrospinal fluid, urine, and other specimens. For most laboratories a centrifuge with a 6 × 15 ml or 8 × 15 ml head is adequate; it should have a variable speed control and a relative centrifugal force of not less than 2300 g, be fitted with a brake, incorporate essential safety features, and be supplied with spare carbon brushes and a clear instruction

Laboratory equipment—where are the tools to do the work?

manual. (A swing out rather than an angled head is preferable, although this may be less readily available and more expensive.)

Hettich Zentrifugen Company manufactures a 12 volt battery operated, variable speed, 6×15 ml angle head centrifuge (EBAIII 2009), price £192. A similar 6×15 ml mains electricity model is also available. The mains model is supplied in the United Kingdom by Arnold Horwell Ltd. One of the lowest priced, small, swing out and angle head variable speed centrifuges, equipped with brake and safety features, is the MLW T51 model available from Clandon Scientific Ltd (fig 2). It costs £310, plus £72·91 for an 8×15 ml swing out head, or £41·96 for a 4×15 ml head. The maximum speed is 2450 g (4200 rpm) for the eight tube head and 2800 g (4500 rpm) for the four tube head. A 24 place, mains operated microhaematocrit centrifuge is available from Hawksley and Sons Ltd, price £265.

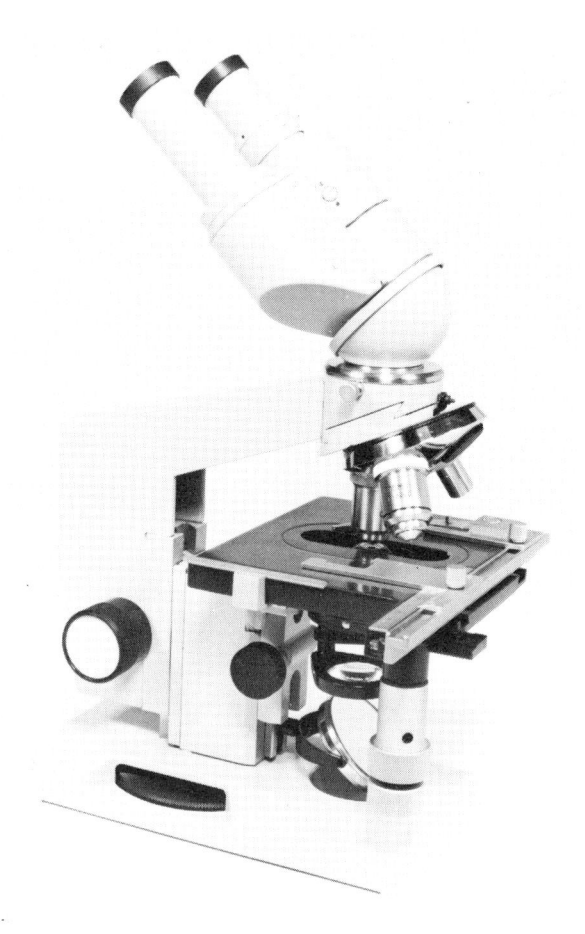

FIG 1—Zenith binocular microscope.

HEAT BLOCK OR WATER BATH

The main use of a heat block or water bath in a district laboratory is for cross matching blood safely. It should be controlled thermostatically and operate from a 12 volt battery and mains electricity supply. A small low priced battery/mains portable heat block/incubator will soon be available from Primary Health Equipment Ltd. The block holds 6×12 mm diameter tubes and 3×16 mm diameter tubes, but individual laboratories may request the size of holes they require if the standard block is not suitable. With the block removed and lid in place, the heating unit functions well as an incubator for keeping specimens warm during transit to the laboratory. The unit will cost about £49·55, complete with block. A transformer to operate the unit from the mains electricity supply will also be available.

HAEMOGLOBIN METER

An ideal haemoglobin meter would be one that is low priced, reliable, accurate, rugged, tropicalised, and capable of operating from inexpensive solar cells or rechargeable batteries (or mains electricity); it should be one that gives a direct readout and does not require the blood to be diluted. The ideal has yet to be designed, but the small Delphi haemoglobin meter (fig 3) fulfils many of these criteria. It gives a direct readout and may be easily calibrated for either the oxyhaemoglobin or cyanmethaemoglobin method. It is rugged and reports from several developing countries have shown it to be reliable. It operates from a 9 volt battery or from a mains electricity supply through a transformer. It is available from Delphi Industries Ltd, priced about £300. A direct readout, compact, battery/mains Hb meter is also available from Buffalo Medical Specialities (BMS) Inc. It is priced about £150, which includes the calibration standards (for cyanmethaemoglobin and oxyhaemoglobin methods) and transformer.

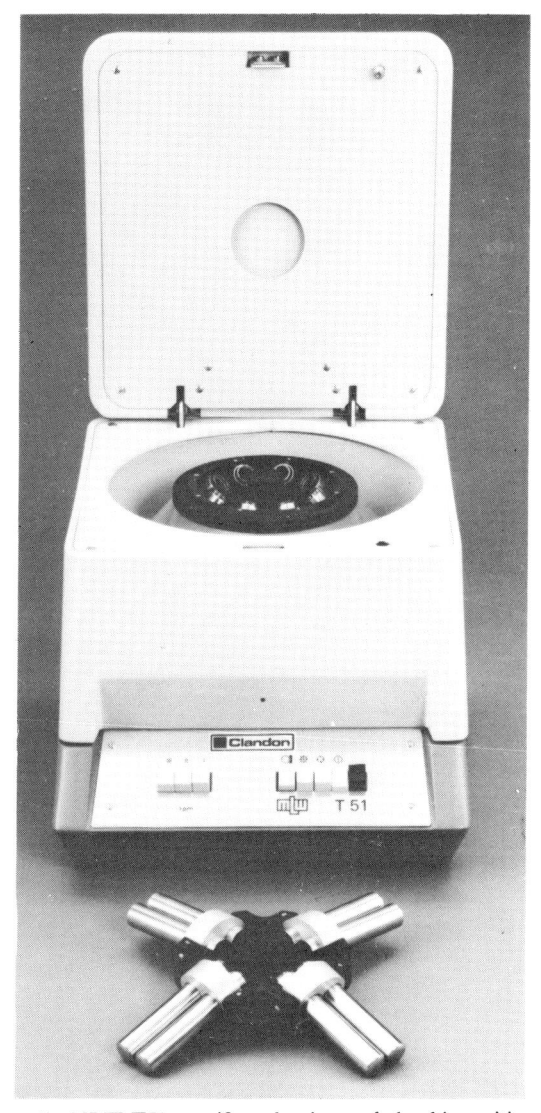

FIG 2—MLW T51 centrifuge showing angle head in position and swing out head for 8×15 ml tubes.

COLORIMETER

The new Model CO 700D medical colorimeter manufactured by Walden Precision Apparatus (WPA) Ltd is highly recommended (fig 4). Because it has been designed for use in developing countries

Laboratory equipment—where are the tools to do the work?

it can be operated from a 12 volt battery or mains electrical supply. It is priced £195, which includes a complete set of integral Ilford filters (No 601–608) covering the wavelength range 400–700 nm with a bandwidth of 40 nm. The filters are specially glass mounted and sealed to protect against fungal growth in humid climates. They are moved into place by turning a clearly marked dial. Being digital and using the latest technology, the CO 700D colorimeter is rugged and easy to operate and maintain by the user. A further advantage is that the sample compartment holds two cuvettes. A pack of cuvettes is supplied with each instrument.

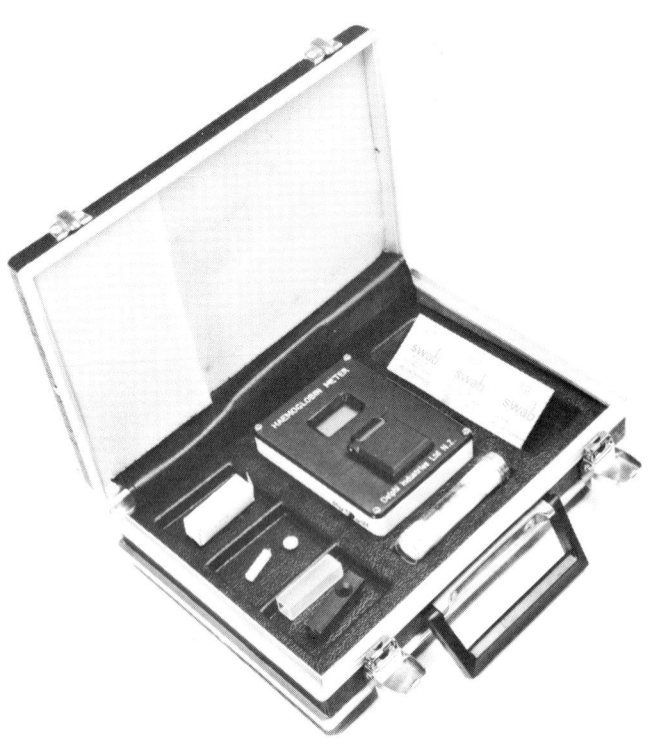

FIG 3—Delphi battery and mains haemoglobin meter with accessories.

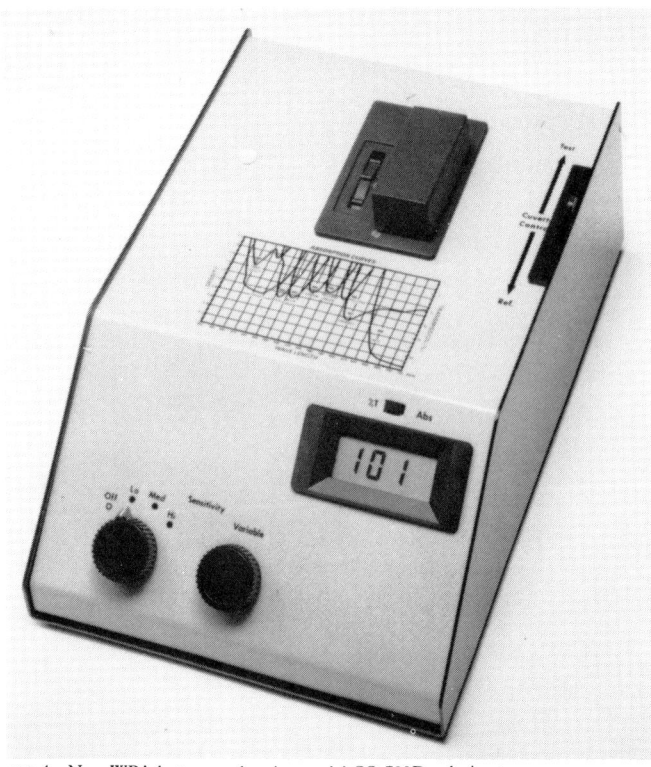

FIG 4—New WPA battery and mains model CO 700D colorimeter.

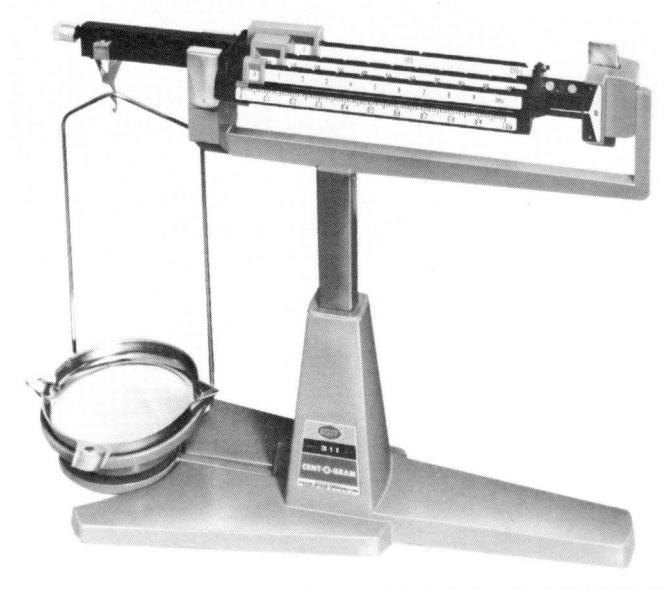

FIG 5—Ohaus balance with 0·01 g sensitivity and 311 g capacity.

WATER STILL

A water still is needed to provide distilled water to make chemical reagents and reference solutions. For preparing water to make stains a simple porcelain filter candle can be used. The pharmacy is likely to need a still to produce pyrogen free water, so it may be possible to share the same still between the two departments. A low cost 3 kW still with a capacity of about 4 l/hour is the Quickfit model W14S, available from J Bibby Science Products Ltd, price £295. It has the advantage of requiring a minimum of cooling water. An automatic cutout operates to prevent overheating if the water supply fails, and there is also a thermal fuse and a preset constant levelling device. The still is easy to clean, and spare parts are readily available. Although the Quickfit still requires mains electricity, sufficient distilled water can usually be made during the hours when the hospital generator is operating.

A new water still for use in developing countries has been designed recently by the Central Scientific Instrument Organisation in India. For details readers should write to the director of the organisation.

STERILISER

In a district hospital the sterilising needs of the laboratory are usually met by the central sterilising supply unit. If, however, the district laboratory is performing culture and sensitivity tests it will require its own autoclave. A range of portable autoclaves that may be operated from mains electricity or a gas or a Primus stove are available from Arnold and Sons Ltd. Six models are available in two sizes: 29 cm diameter × 27 cm depth, and 28 cm diameter × 50 cm depth. They range in price from £149·80 to £501·71. The stand for the gas ring or burner is £21·13. Autoclave control indicator tubes or time steam temperature (TST) strips are available from Albert Browne Ltd.

REFRIGERATOR

A refrigerator is essential for storing reagents, antisera, and some test kits and for preserving patients' sera and other specimens. A separate carefully controlled refrigerator is essential for the safe storage of blood. Gas or kerosene operated refrigerators are required in hospitals without mains electricity.

Laboratory equipment—where are the tools to do the work?

The blood bank refrigerator should be gas operated because the temperature can be better controlled than in a kerosene operated unit. Kerosene and reliable thermostatically gas operated refrigerators are available from Electrolux Ltd. Kerosene refrigerators are available locally in most developing countries.

Product information sheets regarding the specifications and availability of refrigeration units and insulated cold boxes for the transportation of vaccine can be obtained from the Expanded Programme of Immunisation (EPI) Unit, WHO, 1211 Geneva 27, Switzerland. *How to look after a refrigerator* is a concise, easy to understand manual giving instructions for the care and maintenance of kerosene, gas, and electric refrigerators in developing countries. It is available from Appropriate Health Resources and Technologies Acting Group Ltd (AHRTAG).

BALANCE

A balance with a sensitivity of 0·01 g is required in a district laboratory. A trip type balance is also of value for the rapid weighing of stains and chemicals that do not require accurate weighing. The Ohaus balances with integral weights are suitable and inexpensive. The Ohaus model 311 with a sensitivity of 0·01 g and capacity of 311 g (fig 5) costs £98. The Ohaus Havard trip balance with a sensitivity of 0·1 g and capacity of 2000 g costs £97. Both balances are available in the United Kingdom from Gallenkamp and Co Ltd.

INCUBATOR

For laboratories that can carry out culture and sensitivity tests an incubator is required. In the low priced range of incubators that operate from a mains electricity source the Gallenkamp economy incubator model INA-300 size 1 (575 × 590 × 490 mm high) is well insulated and fitted with an inside door and a hydraulic type thermostat. It is available from A Gallenkamp Ltd, price £297. A low priced thermal plastic 12 volt battery or mains incubator 444 × 368 × 444 mm high is available from GQF Manufacturing Company, priced about $180.

Conclusion

Appropriate equipment for use in the district hospital laboratory in developing countries is urgently needed. Such equipment must be designed according to medical needs and the surroundings in which it will be used. It must be reliable, robust, and easy to use by those with a limited technical background. It must also be produced at a price that such countries can afford. Much redesigning, training, sharing of resources, and transfer of technology to developing countries are needed if the majority of the world's sick are to have access to investigations essential to diagnosis and the major communicable diseases are to be controlled.

References

[1] Cheesbrough M. *Medical laboratory manual for tropical countries.* Volume 1, 1981; volume 2, 1984. Tropical Health Technology Ltd, 14 Bevills Close, Doddington, Cambridgeshire PE15 0TT, UK. The manuals are produced on a low cost basis to assist developing countries.
[2] World Health Organisation. *Specifications for production and/or assembly of basic laboratory equipment.* Geneva: WHO, 1983.
[3] World Health Organisation. *Supply, maintenance and repair of health care laboratory equipment in developing countries.* Geneva: WHO, 1983. (LAB/83.8.)

Manufacturers

Primary Health Equipment Ltd, 365 Eastfield Road, Peterborough, Cambs PE1 4RD, UK. The company was formed and is managed by Mr Alan Riley, a qualified design engineer and member of the consultative group for appropriate technology in the field of health laboratory technology.

McArthur Microscopes Ltd, Landbeach, Cambridge, Cambs CB4 4ED, UK.

Hettich Zentrifugen, Andreas Hettich, Postfach 4255, D-7200 Tuttingen, West Germany.

Delphi Industries Ltd, 27 Ben Lomond Crescent, Pakuranga, Auckland, New Zealand.

Buffalo Medical Specialities Mfg Inc., 3110B 44 Ave. North, St Petersburg, Fl 33714, USA.

Clandon Scientific Ltd, Lyson's Avenue, Ash Vale, Aldershot, Hampshire GU12 5QR, UK.

Hawksley and Sons Ltd, 12 Peter Road, Lancing, Sussex.

Walden Precision Apparatus Ltd, The Old Station, Linton, Cambridge CB1 6NW, UK.

J Bibby Science Products Ltd, Tilling Drive, Walton, Stone, Staffordshire ST15 0SA, UK.

Central Scientific Instrument Organisation, Chandigarh, India.

Arnold and Sons Ltd, Bentalls, Basildon, Essex SS14 3BY, UK.

Albert Brown Ltd, Chancery House, Abbey Gate, Leicester LE4 0AA, UK.

Electrolux AB, International Division, S-10545, Stockholm, Sweden.

AHRTAG, 85 Marylebone High Street, London, W1M 3DE, UK.

A Gallenkamp Ltd, PO Box 290, Technico House, Christopher Street, London EC2P 2ER, UK.

GQF Manufacturing Company, PO Box 1552, Savannah, Ga 31402, USA.

EQUIPMENT FOR THE GASTROENTEROLOGIST

JOHN NICHOLLS

In Western countries gastroenterologists depend to a great extent on supporting services: radiology, biochemistry, haematology, microbiology, and histopathology. In the Third World, where these support services may be rudimentary or even non-existent, the gastroenterologist must learn to make full use of his own facilities and to extend his skills by undertaking some of the techniques that he would normally delegate to others.

Basic needs

Before consideration of the tools of the trade it is worth emphasising that a good history is always important, and as local interpretation of common terms such as indigestion, colic, and bellyache vary from country to country or even district to district it is a good idea to compile a glossary of local terms. One of the best ways to do this is to enlist the help of a locally trained community nurse. Her translating skills are likely to be invaluable and should be sought early, before misconceptions in the ability to acquire knowledge of a local dialect delude the patients (and the doctor) that the practitioner is fully conversant with the local vernacular.

Over the past few years Western doctors have been spoilt by ready access to disposable items, largely because of the high labour costs concerned in making such items reusable. Where labour is cheap, however, certain items such as mouth spatulas, rubber gloves, syringes, needles, and proctoscopes may have to be reused. The main disadvantage of reusable items is that there is a risk of transmitting infection including viral hepatitis if sterilisation is not adequate. In terms of cost, reusable items are usually cheaper in the long run.

Proctoscopes and sigmoidoscopes are the basic items of equipment, and I think that an interchangeable set with a fibre light source—for example, the Lloyd Davies pattern, supplied by Seward, UAC House, Blackfriars Road, London SE1 9UG—is preferable to the newer disposable apparatus. To use these instruments effectively a good light is essential, and fibreoptic bundles are robust enough to withstand long use. The bulb for the light source may be obtained from a local photographic dealer. This source of light is much better and more reliable than that obtained from a battery or transformer. Although a good strong torch is adequate for proctoscopy in areas where the electricity supply is unreliable, it is inadequate for sigmoidoscopy, so in the long run the fibreoptic bundle is the best bet.

A glass Gabriel syringe and supply of reusable needles are further pieces of essential equipment. These enable the gastroenterologist to treat piles—a surprisingly common complaint in the Third World—in the outpatient department.

Good weighing scales—for example, the basic model supplied by Marsden, 388 Harrow Road, London W9—which also measure height are another useful item. Finally, a tape measure and pair of Holtain skin callipers are useful to assess malnutrition. It is a good idea to measure a range of normal people in the community to establish a rough estimate of local standards.

Special equipment

Many of the following items rely on electricity, and even if there is a fairly reliable mains supply it is advisable to have a small portable petrol driven generator.

A microscope is essential, and the gastroenterologist must learn to use this proficiently. It is advisable to have a microscope in or near the outpatient department so that rapid microscopy of specimens of stools for parasites and of urine for casts and cells may be carried out. The microscope should be capable of up to 400 times magnification. Those that are suitable for this—for example, a Leitz microscope—usually operate with internal illumination only; thus it is advisable to keep a second microscope that is illuminated by natural light in case the electricity supply fails. The microscope may require to be tropicalised to prevent fungus growing on the lenses in humid environments. The same microscope may be used to examine blood samples to assess red cell morphology and for looking at thick films for malarial parasites. A supply of counting chambers and appropriate stains (Giemsa rather than Leishman) must, therefore, be supplied, and an oil immersion lens of 100 times magnification.

The inequality between Western and Third World countries is possibly nowhere more apparent than in the laboratory. Automated instruments and computers have little or no place in the Third World.[1] I have compiled a brief guide to what equipment is needed and which investigations the gastroenterologist may expect (or arrange) to be obtained simply and cheaply:

(1) Refrigerator: for general purposes, and for keeping vaccines, reagents, etc.

(2) Microscope (as above).

(3) Simple colorimeter: this needs to be cheap, sturdy, and capable of operating trouble free in extremes of climate. With this, measurement of urea, bilirubin, alkaline phosphatase, calcium, and protein concentrations is possible.

(4) A local supply of chemistry systems: if these are not available the stick test strips (Miles-Ames) are preferable to prepacked chemistry systems.

(5) Flame photometer: this requires a gas supply in addition to electricity but is more robust than the ion selective electrode apparatus, which requires only electricity. It enables sodium and potassium concentrations to be measured.

From this list evidently the scope of laboratory investigations is necessarily restricted; investigation of complex metabolic problems is likely, therefore, to be beyond the means of the gastroenterologist in the Third World. The World Health

Organisation has prepared a manual with detailed descriptions of essential tests for the primary hospital in the Third World.[2]

Providing an endoscopy service

In developed countries endoscopy is an essential part of gastroenterological practice, both in diagnosis and, increasingly, in treatment. But is this technology appropriate for the Third World? I believe that it is, and if the equipment is chosen carefully the gastroenterologist may provide an effective endoscopy service, even in a fairly primitive environment. Difficulties in funding the capital cost of an endoscopic service should be weighed against the possible savings in other departments—for example, the x ray department and operating theatre. Maintenance of the endoscope and repair costs need to be kept to a minimum by careful handling (restricted to the expert user), scrupulous cleaning, and possibly some patient selection (a young alcoholic may destroy a fibre bundle with one bite). Another potential hazard of providing an endoscopy service is that of transmitting the hepatitis virus. In developing countries the reservoir of asymptomatic carriers may be high, and thus the risk is proportionately increased. It is, therefore, important to follow the guidelines on disinfection of endoscopes given by the endoscopy subcommittee of the British Society of Gastroenterology.[3]

Everyone will have experienced the frustration of attempting to use a particular piece of equipment only to find that the vital connector, plug, or fuse is not available. The frustration is likely to be heightened if it takes weeks to obtain the missing part. To avoid this the endoscopist must buy a comprehensive, adaptable, and interchangeable system of endoscopes. It is thus advisable to purchase equipment produced by one company alone, despite the claims by manufacturers of the individual uniqueness of their product. The two companies that deal with the most comprehensive range of endoscopic equipment in the United Kingdom are KeyMed (KeyMed House, Stock Road, Southend-on-Sea, Essex), who supply the Olympus range, and Pyser (102 College Road, Harrow HA1 1BQ), who supply the Fuji range. I suggest that an end viewing gastroduodenoscope and a colonoscope are purchased as the two basic pieces of equipment, together with biopsy facilities and possibly snares. (The snares may require modification to be used with a standard diathermy apparatus.) Refinements of these endoscopes for investigating the pancreatic and biliary trees are not usually an advantage because treatment is likely to be so difficult that it cannot be undertaken readily in a Third World hospital.

Providing an endoscopy service has the obvious advantage that the endoscopist will not have to rely on a radiological colleague for barium examination. Provided that the gastroenterologist becomes proficient at using the microscope he may manage without a specialist in pathology, for many pathological specimens may be identified by their macroscopic appearance alone. Biopsy specimens are suitably small to be sent away by post, so it may be useful to establish a link with a laboratory in the United Kingdom that is prepared to report on the histological appearance of such specimens whenever necessary.

In this speciality the link with an interested pathologist can be fruitful. Many gastroenterologists use jejunal biopsy via a Crosby capsule in their assessment of small bowel function. Local conditions may affect the appearance of the small bowel mucosa in such a way that diagnosis may be difficult. The use of a Crosby capsule in the Third World may not be possible because of the skill required; and the problem may be overcome by using endoscopic biopsy specimens taken from the third part of the duodenum.

Additional items

Various needles may be used for percutaneous biopsy: Tru-cut or Menghini needles are available from the American Hospital Supply, Station Road, Didcot, Oxfordshire. These needles, however, are expensive because they are disposable, and the pathological specimen that is obtained is small and will almost certainly have to be sent away to a laboratory that is familiar with handling cores of tissue. Pathological specimens of tissue may, of course, be obtained at laparoscopy, but this technique demands experience and you also need expensive apparatus and a supply of carbon dioxide gas. As a rule, open biopsy at operation is more satisfactory, and it gives the surgeon the opportunity to assess the full extent of the disease and, if possible, to treat.

Special therapeutic equipment will not necessarily differ from that used in Western countries, although certain adaptations may be required to meet local needs. Stoma care equipment does not need modification as the bags are designed to cope with a wide range of circumstances. Companies with a comprehensive range of products are: Abbot Laboratories Ltd, Queensborough, Kent; Colopast Ltd, Bridge House, Orchard Lane, Huntingdon, Cambridge; Downs Surgical, Church Path, Mitcham, Surrey; Squibb Surgicare Ltd, Squibb House, 141 Staines Road, Hounslow, Middlesex.

It is always important to find out what the home conditions of the patient are like: lack of a good water supply or an adequate drainage system leads to obvious problems in terms of maintaining personal hygiene and disposing of plastic materials. It is equally important to be aware that local customs may result in a patient with a stoma becoming ostracised. These factors should influence your decision to operate—for example, on a patient with abdominal cancer—and leave the patient with a colostomy or ileostomy. Remember that heroic attempts to remove cancer are not greeted with the same enthusiasm as in the West. An international organisation of stomatherapists (World Council of Enterostomal Therapists, 926 East Tallmadge Avenue, Suite C, Akron, Ohio 44310, USA) has been formed to help with stoma problems world wide.

Parenteral nutrition is seldom practicable. Even if it were possible to set up and satisfactorily maintain a long intravenous line the preparation of suitable solutions for infusion, ensuring their sterility, and monitoring their effect will demand too much in terms of time and resources. Although malnutrition is a common problem, it may, in most cases, be treated by oral supplements or by feeding the patient through a fine bore feeding catheter. A range of these catheters is supplied by Britannia Pharmaceuticals Ltd, 7-11 High Street, Reigate, Surrey RH2 9RR. These tubes are quite difficult to pass, and if they cannot be obtained readily a standard Ryle's tube, which is usually well tolerated by the patient, should suffice.

The gastroenterologist's prescribing habits will be influenced by the prevalence of infective diseases of the gastrointestinal tract. Thus antiparasitic agents, antibiotics, antidiarrhoeals, and antiemetics are essential. Constipation is a common complaint despite bulky diets, and therefore a choice of simple aperients or local laxative medicines is useful. The choice of drug must be tempered by cost, by its effectiveness, and by patient compliance. This applies particularly to compounds such as H_2 receptor antagonists, steroids, and antispasmodics. Patients who may be expected to remain on long term treatment cannot necessarily either obtain or afford this. Under such circumstances surgery may have to be performed as a realistic alternative to long term drug treatment. The demand for medicine or tablets is often great; many patients attending the outpatient clinic will not be satisfied unless they are provided with tangible evidence of illness and treatment. Thus in my view a low cost placebo may be useful—either a Western proprietary medicine or one based on a traditional medicine.

The merit of giving hepatitis B vaccine is a wide issue but is one in which the gastroenterologist may get concerned, and he may be expected to advise the local health ministry before it embarks on an expensive vaccination programme. He may also have to advise on preventive measures—for example, how to organise a clean water supply, dispose of sewage, etc. Thus he may be expected to undertake tasks outside his normal skills, and stripped of ancillary services the gastroenterologist faces a number of challenges. To meet these there is nothing more effective than enthusiasm, flexibility, and the application of knowledge in an appropriate manner. After all, this costs little apart from commitment and a sense of purpose, and in turn it may be rewarded richly.

I thank Dr L Farrow and Dr D Burnett for help in the preparation of this paper, and Mrs C Surrey for typing the manuscript.

References

[1] Mitchell FL. Comparison between problems on instrumentation in developed and developing countries. *First African and Mediterranean congress of clinical chemistry*. Milan: Italian Society of Clinical Biochemistry, 1980:49-53.

[2] Mitchell FL. Supply, maintenance and repair of health care laboratory equipment in developing countries. *Clinical Chemistry newsletter; news from African, Mediterranean and Near East countries* 1983;4:142-55.

[3] Cotton PB, Williams CB. *Practical gastrointestinal endoscopy*. Oxford: Blackwell, 1980.

THE CARDIOLOGIST IN THE THIRD WORLD

E G L WILKINS, J I G STRANG

Unlike his contemporaries in developed countries, the cardiologist in the Third World needs to adapt his specialised knowledge to compensate for the absence of sophisticated equipment, trained staff, and expensive drugs. He must make full use of the information obtained from the history, clinical examination, and basic investigations and must learn to manage with a small number of inexpensive drugs which are available locally. In addition, he may have to develop a working proficiency in allied disciplines such as radiology and pathology. By such practice he should be able to diagnose and manage most cardiac conditions. This article is based on our experience of working in Umtata Hospital, which is the referral centre for Transkei (in southern Africa), a country with a population of three million where the prevailing diseases—rheumatic heart disease, tuberculous pericarditis, hypertension, and dilated cardiomyopathy—are similar to those encountered in many developing countries. We are general physicians with an interest in cardiology and believe that in many developing countries the cardiologist is more likely to be a general physician than a specialist. The establishment of cardiac surgery in Umtata is a measure of our interest.

Patients in developing countries often present late, with advanced disease and obvious clinical signs that may enable the clinician to make a diagnosis without recourse to investigations. A knowledge of the prevailing diseases in the area is important and may best be obtained by reference to local publications, since descriptions of disease in Western texts are not always applicable to a developing country.

Equipment

When buying equipment it is important to ensure that an after sales service, with a supply of major spare parts, is guaranteed. It is a good idea to order spares when the equipment is purchased because normal wear and tear will necessitate replacement of certain minor parts—for example, rubber limb cuffs of an electrocardiograph, stethoscope tubing and ear pieces, ophthalmoscope bulbs, etc. The addresses of the companies listed at the end of this article are the head offices in Britain, but they will be able to provide information about overseas services.

A good stethoscope is essential; this should have a bell and diaphragm preferably incorporated in one piece—for example, the Littmann combination. Mercury sphygmomanometers (such as the Accoson model 125) with solid cases and folding lids are more robust than anaeroid devices and easier to repair. In addition to the standard adult cuff, a larger cuff for obese adults and a smaller cuff for children and thin adults should be available. Wrap around bandage cuffs are more durable than Velcro or hook ones. A sturdy, battery operated interchangeable ophthalmoscope and auroscope is useful, particularly if it may be used with rechargeable batteries. The Welch Allyn 3·5 V halogen diagnostic set, supplied with charger unit, from Seward Medical is a good example. Assessment of fluid balance by change of weight is usually more reliable than trying to keep accurate fluid balance charts, so a good set of weighing scales is necessary.

In the laboratory

Simple equipment such as a fridge, microscope, staining reagents, and colorimeter allow basic laboratory tests to be carried out that help to provide circumstantial evidence of cardiac disease—for example, leucocytosis, anaemia, microscopic haematuria, uraemia, etc. If the facilities for bacteriological culture are not available Gram or Ziehl-Neelsen staining of pus or sputum may identify the causative organism, and this simple test may be done by the doctor. When it is possible to forward blood culture bottles to a nearby laboratory for processing a supply should be kept for patients with suspected infective endocarditis.

The antistreptolysin O titre and Venereal Disease Research Laboratory test are important in the diagnosis of rheumatic fever and cardiovascular syphilis. They may be measured with simple and inexpensive kits such as those obtainable from Wellcome Reagents Ltd. Similar kits are available for the measurement of prothrombin time (Ortho Diagnostics Ltd).

X ray equipment

In many hospitals the *x* ray equipment is the most valuable piece of equipment—and the one that is most easily, and frequently, rendered inoperable. Because of this the cardiologist should have a working knowledge of the machinery and also be able to take, and therefore instruct others in taking, a posteroanterior chest film of adequate diagnostic quality. (The details and specifications of *x* ray equipment have been discussed in the article by PES Palmer (p 9)).

A radiograph of the chest gives information about heart size, enlargement of the chambers, the pulmonary circulation, and coexistent parenchymal lung disease (fig 1). In the absence of specialised techniques to demonstrate mitral valve calcification a penetrated left lateral *x* ray film is helpful. Where there are facilities for fluoroscopy and barium swallow these may provide additional information to assess the suitability of a patient for closed mitral valvotomy.

The electrocardiograph

The single channel Fukuda FJC 1000 is a cheap, robust, and reliable machine that is easy to operate. Although this particular

The cardiologist in the Third World

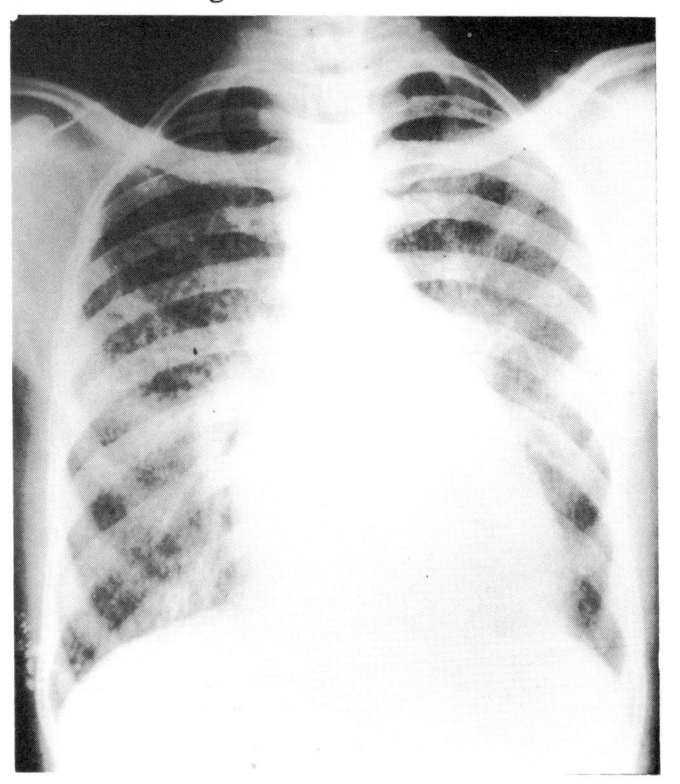

FIG 1—In mitral valve disease it may be difficult to distinguish secondary pulmonary haemosiderosis from active or inactive tuberculosis. In ill patients or when contemplating surgery, it may be necessary to give a therapeutic trial or operative cover with antituberculous drugs.

model has been discontinued, the Fukuda Denshi FK-11 (Cardiacare Instruments (UK) Ltd) is very similar and can run off the mains or a rechargeable battery, dry cell batteries, or a car battery. Standard lubricant jellies,[1] or even tap water,[2] may be used instead of expensive electrode jelly.

Before ascribing any abnormal tracing to underlying heart disease the physician must be familiar with the patterns of normal variants. These are usually ST segment and T wave changes, which may occur in otherwise healthy black people[3] and may be confused with patterns seen in conditions such as acute pericarditis. The tracing invariably becomes normal after exercise.[4] An electrocardiogram is also useful in the detection of hypokalaemia and hyperkalaemia if a flame photometer to measure plasma potassium concentrations is not available.

Specialist equipment

If the hospital has facilities for cardiac surgery echocardiography is helpful in deciding which patients would benefit most from surgery. Although M mode echocardiography provides information about cardiac function as well as structure—and may thus obviate the need for cardiac catheterisation[5]—two dimensional echocardiography is simpler to use. (It may also be used by other specialists, such as obstetricians.) We use an ATL 100 sector scanner (Squibb Medical Systems Ltd) and find that it saves time and unnecessary investigation with less informative tests (fig 2). With this machine the physician can confirm, or refute, the presence of a mobile noncalcific valve in mitral stenosis and detect the presence of left atrial thrombus. It is also helpful in the diagnosis of infective endocarditis and the investigation of heart failure or cardiomegaly of unknown cause. We have found it particularly helpful in differentiating cor pulmonale, dilated cardiomyopathy, occult valvular disease, pericardial effusion, and constrictive pericarditis.

A spare scan head should be ordered when buying the machine, and it is worth knowing how to remove the keyboard in case it develops a fault, as paying for a company engineer to travel to the machine will add to the expense of repairs. If cardiac surgery is undertaken a simple cardiac monitor and a defibrillator should be available. We use a portable DC defibrillator with a built in monitor (Philips B D 500, now replaced by the Philips E D 420; Honeywell Medical Electronics Division) for operative and postoperative monitoring. It is unusual to see patients with ischaemic heart disease, so the defibrillator is rarely required after a cardiac arrest due to ventricular fibrillation. Conditions requiring cardiac pacing are similarly uncommon, and so, if necessary, patients are referred to a centre in neighbouring South Africa.

Management of patients

Drug regimens must take into account the fact that many hospitals in the Third World have limited resources and that patient compliance may be poor. Characteristics that are important in deciding which drug to use include low cost, availability, once daily dosage, and patient acceptability. Additional measures—for example, weight reduction and reduction of salt intake in the treatment of hypertension—may be worth trying but are often impractical because of the patient's way of life. We base our treatment on the following selection of drugs: digoxin, a thiazide and loop diuretic, a vasodilator such as hydralazine, hypotensive drugs such as reserpine and methyldopa, emergency trolley drugs (adrenaline, atropine, and calcium), anticoagulants and aspirin, penicillin, and four antituberculosis

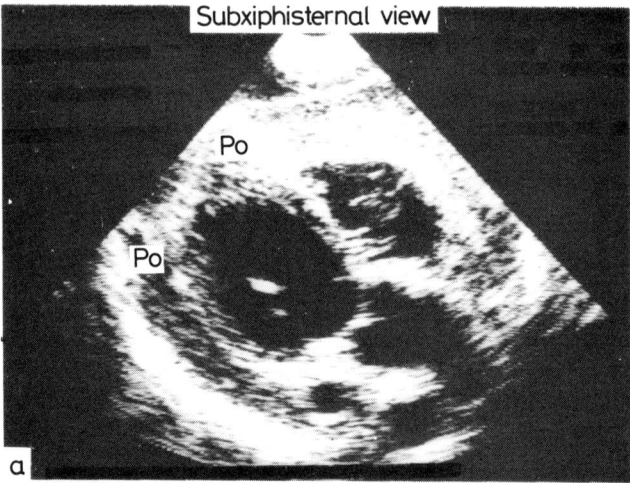

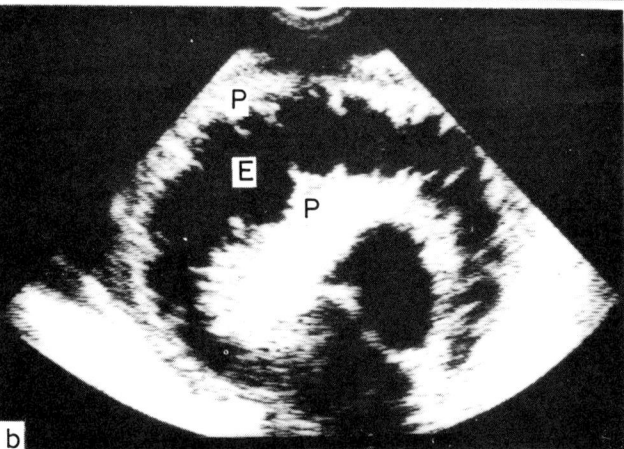

FIG 2—(a) Subacute constrictive pericarditis showing thick fibrocaseous inflammatory tissue (Po="porridge") in the pericardial sac of a man who presented with congestive cardiac failure of unknown cause. Surgery is unlikely to help at this stage because this tissue cannot be adequately stripped. (b) Moderately large pericardial effusion (E) with thickened visceral and parietal pericardium (P): many fibrinous strands can be seen. Pericardiocentesis may not help the haemodynamic abnormality which is due to visceral constriction.

The cardiologist in the Third World

agents including streptomycin, isoniazid, and pyrazinamide. Morphine, salbutamol, and chlorpromazine[6] have useful cardiovascular effects, and these three are also stocked. These drugs provide effective treatment for cardiac failure and hypertension, treatment and prophylaxis of rheumatic fever and bacterial endocarditis, treatment of tuberculous pericarditis, and the essentials for dealing with cardiac emergencies. Thiazide diuretics are the best first line treatment for hypertension in southern Africa,[7] and this coupled with the infrequency of ischaemic heart disease explains the absence of β blockers from the list.

An intravenous infusion of salbutamol (10 mg salbutamol in 200 ml 5% dextrose) given eight hourly is used to treat patients with refractory cardiac failure. It is safe and easy to monitor, and the most important side effect—hypokalaemia—can be anticipated. Our need for antiarrhythmic drugs is limited because the only arrhythmia that we commonly see is atrial fibrillation, which may be controlled with digoxin. If reversion to sinus rhythm is likely to be successful quinidine is used.

Thromboembolism complicating heart disease is an important cause of morbidity and mortality and so heparin and warfarin must be available. It may be impossible to monitor anticoagulation—for example, if a patient comes from a remote area—and in this instance we prescribe either warfarin 5 mg or aspirin 300 mg daily. While not ideal, this is part of the reality of a developing country.

The most effective prophylaxis against recurrent rheumatic fever is intramuscular benzathine penicillin 1·2 megaunits monthly.[8] Infective endocarditis may be treated simply and usually successfully with the combination of penicillin and streptomycin. Ideally rifampicin should be included in any treatment regimen for tuberculosis but is expensive and may be difficult to obtain. In its absence triple and preferably quadruple initial treatment is advisable.

Cardiac surgery

In our practice the only operations that can be undertaken safely and give good results are closed mitral valvotomy, pericardiectomy, and ligation of a patent ductus arteriosus. Apart from a rib spreader, periosteal elevator, and Tubbs transventricular dilator (available from Thackray's), no specialised equipment is necessary. We obtained two Tubbs dilators from friends at cardiothoracic centres in Britain and recommend such places as a source of equipment. Despite a need for valvular replacement surgery it cannot be considered a priority because of its high cost, the frequent necessity for further replacement of the valve in children,[9] and the difficulties of postoperative follow up. On the rare occasions when ischaemic heart disease occurs and requires surgery the patient usually belongs to a section of society that can afford to send him to an appropriate centre for treatment. Over the past eight years 110 patients with a clinical diagnosis of constructive pericarditis supported by a compatible chest x ray film and electrocardiogram have been referred for pericardiectomy. In every case the diagnosis was confirmed at operation.

Pericardiocentesis may be performed safely using an intravenous plastic cannula with integral chamber that fills immediately on striking fluid. The metal trocar is then removed and aspiration continued through the relatively soft plastic cannula (fig 3). Myocardial biopsy may establish a specific cause of heart muscle disease, but in the absence of effective treatment for most of these conditions this investigation is of limited use. Biopsy of the pericardium in the presence of an effusion may be helpful and may be performed with standard surgical equipment. Although biopsy specimens may have to be sent away for examination, a tissue diagnosis is usually definitive, so in the long run it may be cheaper and quicker than carrying out less invasive investigations. (A histopathology service for developing countries has been established in London at the department of morbid anatomy, School of Medicine, University College London, University Street, London WC1: contact Dr S Lucas for information.)

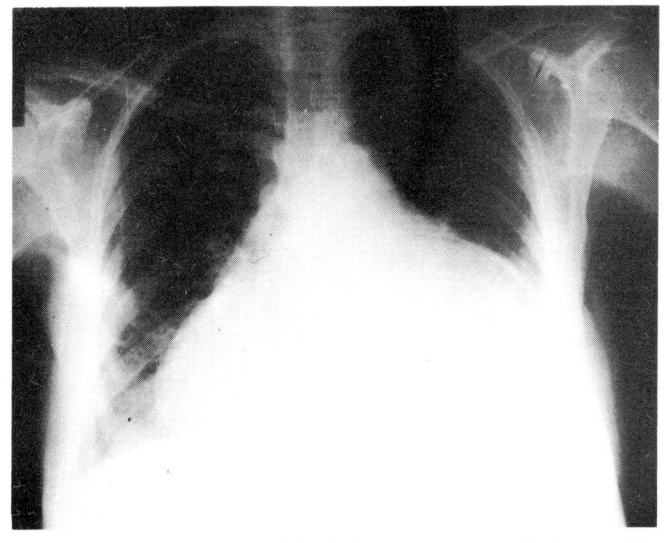

FIG 3—In most cases a pericardial effusion can be confidently diagnosed by clinical examination supported by typical changes on the chest x ray and electrocardiogram. Pericardiocentesis is best performed via the subxiphisternal route, avoiding the pleura and entering the most dependent part of the sac.

Conclusion

Thus with a minimum of equipment and drugs the cardiologist may reduce the impact of cardiovascular disease, which is a major cause of morbidity and mortality in the Third World. Provision of cardiological care must also include the effective application of medical resources to reduce the incidence of cardiovascular disease. The feasibility and effectiveness of a community programme in the control of rheumatic heart disease have been shown,[10] and similar benefits may be expected from the community control of tuberculosis. Recent advances in the production of an antistreptococcal vaccine are encouraging and if successful could lead to the elimination of rheumatic heart disease.[11]

We thank Mr David Mugwanya for help and advice, Dr Derek Gibson of the Brompton Hospital for ultrasound instruction, and colleagues at Wentworth Hospital in Durban.

References

[1] Anonymous. No more jelly? [Editorial.] *Lancet* 1965;i:795-6.
[2] Martin A, Tiernan R, D'Arcy M, O'Brien E. Tap water instead of electrode jelly for electrocardiographic recording. *Br Med J* 1979;i:454.
[3] Krikler DM. The electrocardiogram. *Cardiovascular disease in the tropics.* London: British Medical Association, 1974:160-71.
[4] Przybojewski JZ, Heyns MH, Goldsmith P. Peculiarities of the electrocardiogram in the black population. *Symposium on cardiology in a tropical environment.* Tygerberg, South Africa: South African Medical Research Council, 1982:249-57.
[5] Sutton MG St J, Sutton M St J, Oldershaw P, et al. Valve replacement without preoperative cardiac catheterisation. *N Engl J Med* 1981;305:1233-8.
[6] Young RJ, Lawson AAH, Malone DNS. Treatment of severe hypertension with chlorpromazine and frusemide. *Br Med J* 1980;i:1579.
[7] Seedat YK. Trial of atenolol and chlorthalidone for hypertension in black South Africans. *Br Med J* 1980;281:1241-3.
[8] Markowitz M. Prevention of acute rheumatic fever and rheumatic heart disease. *Preventive cardiology.* London: Butterworths, 1983:47-61.
[9] le Roux BT. Surgery in children with chronic rheumatic heart disease: where are we going? *Symposium on cardiology in a tropical environment.* Tygerberg, South Africa: South African Medical Research Council, 1982:178-80.
[10] Strasser T, Dondog N, El Kholy A, et al. The community control of rheumatic fever and rheumatic heart disease: report of a WHO international cooperative project. *Bull WHO* 1981;59:285-94.
[11] Beachey EH. Can rheumatic heart disease be eliminated? *Symposium on cardiology in a tropical environment.* Tygerberg, South Africa: South African Medical Research Council, 1982:162-70.

Companies listed in article

Accoson, A C Cossor and Sons (Surgical) Ltd, Accoson Works, Vale Road, London N4 1PS.
Cardiacare Instruments (UK) Ltd, 882 Eastern Avenue, Newbury Park, Ilford, Essex IG2 7HY.
Honeywell Medical Electronics Division, Honeywell House, Charles Square, Bracknell, Berkshire RG1 1EB.
Littmann, 3M House, PO Box 1, Bracknell, Berkshire RG12 1JU.
Ortho Diagnostics Systems Ltd, Denmark House, Denmark Street, High Wycombe, Buckinghamshire HP11 2ER.
Seward Medical, 31 New Cavendish Street, London W1M 7RL.
Squibb Medical Systems Ltd, Blackhorse Road, Letchworth, Hertfordshire SG6 1HL.
Thackray's, 69 Weymouth Street, London W1.
Wellcome Reagents Ltd, Temple Hill, Dartford DA1 5AH.

THE RESPIRATORY PHYSICIAN IN A THIRD WORLD DISTRICT HOSPITAL

JOHN MACFARLANE

Respiratory diseases are the commonest cause of hospital attendance and also death in many parts of the Third World. They resulted in 22% of adult admissions to one hospital in Uganda,[1] 23·5% of paediatric admissions in Zambia,[2] and up to 25% of all hospital cases in Papua New Guinea.[3] Respiratory infections, particularly pneumonia and tuberculosis, are the most common conditions, but asthma and non-infectious chronic lung diseases are also common in some areas.[3] Nearly half of the patients seen with a respiratory illness at a medical centre in the southern Maldives were diagnosed as having asthma.[4] After pulmonary tuberculosis, asthma was found to be the most common chronic chest disease in African children in Ibadan, Nigeria.[5]

Thus the main workload of a physician with an interest in respiratory medicine working in a district hospital in the Third World includes pneumonia and its complications such as empyema and lung abscess, other acute respiratory infections, pulmonary tuberculosis, asthma, and (to a lesser extent) other chronic lung disorders. Most of these can be managed without recourse to expensive or complex equipment (table).

Respiratory infections

Respiratory infections are common, and acute pneumonia is responsible for many paediatric and adult admissions. Many patients will not have received antibiotics before they present to the hospital, so a Gram stain of the sputum and sputum culture will often be helpful. A side room equipped with Gram stain kit, slides, and a microscope permits immediate examination of sputum and may also be useful for examining samples of urine and cerebrospinal fluid. Blood cultures should always be taken. Most pneumonias are caused by pneumococcal infections and will respond to simple, cheap antibiotics such as penicillin and ampicillin.[6][7]

Most physicians with an interest in respiratory medicine will adopt the role of the tuberculosis doctor. Many district hospitals have a separate tuberculosis ward or annexe, and a special clinic should be organised if this is not already available. This is helpful because it provides the opportunity to train nurses and interpreters to manage and educate patients with tuberculosis (fig 1). Many patients have little idea of the duration of their illness, but occasionally help will be obtained by, for example, gauging the age of cuts performed by the local doctor (fig 2). Useful advice on organising a tuberculosis service is given in a book by King.[8] Diagnosis depends on the appearance of the chest radiograph and examination of the sputum for tubercle bacilli. Facilities for culture of the tubercle bacilli may not be available, so if there is no information about the local pattern of sensitivity of *Mycobacterium tuberculosis* to drugs it is a good idea to send a consecutive series of smear positive sputum samples to the nearest laboratory that can undertake culture and sensitivity testing. If only a small number of patients are seen Ziehl-Neelsen staining of fresh samples of sputum may be carried out in the clinic. Larger numbers may warrant the use of fluorescence microscopy in the hospital's laboratory.

Tuberculin skin testing is of little diagnostic value in teenagers and adults but aids diagnosis in children and is helpful for checking the immunity of staff working closely with patients with tuberculosis. A Heaf gun and Evans undiluted purified protein derivative (shelf life three years at 4°C) is a well tried method for the skin tests.[8] The end of the Heaf gun should be soaked in spirit and flamed between each use, or the end plate may be changed on the magnetic version.

Drug treatment will depend on what is available locally, but, if possible, the standard guidelines of modern antituberculosis chemotherapy should be followed.[9][10] Ideally, treatment protocols should be agreed on nationally to minimise problems with drug resistance and to allow bulk purchasing to reduce costs. Regular

Details of special equipment mentioned in text

	Approximate price in United Kingdom (excluding VAT)	United Kingdom supplier
Heaf multiple puncture gun Mark 5	54·30	Eschmann Bros and Walsh Ltd, Peter Road, Lancing, West Sussex BN16 8TJ
(20 spare needles)	8·05	
Heaf multiple puncture gun Mark 7 with magnetic head	43·45	"
(spare 6 point plates, box of 50)	17·10	
Wright peak flow meter	180·00	Clement Clarke International Ltd, 15 Wigmore Street, London W1H 9LA
Standard Wright mini peak flow meter	9·96	"
(spare plastic sterilisable mouthpieces)	0·40	
Vitalograph R model spirometer	550·00	Vitalograph Medical Instrumentation, Maids Moreton House, Buckingham MK18 1SW
(200 spare recording charts)	13·00	
Porta-Peak peak flow gauge	30·00	Medic-Aid Ltd, Hooks Lane, Pegham, Sussex PO21 3PP
Porta-Neb 50 Multivolt nebuliser pump	86·50	"
Aerolyser electric nebuliser pump CFIR	119·69	Aerosol Products Ltd, 680 Garratt Lane, London SW17 0NP
Intersurgical nebuliser chamber + tubing (supplied in boxes of 20)	0·93 each	Intersurgical Ltd, Charwell House, Lincoln Way, Sunbury on Thames, Middlesex TW16 7HJ
Abrams pleural biopsy needle with 3 way tap (ref 3030)	35·30	NI Medical Ltd, PO Box 3, 26 Thornhill Road, Redditch B98 9NL
Trocar and cannula for intercostal tube insertion	18·39	Rocket of London, Imperial Way, Watford WD2 4XX
Roberts suction pump	237·82	GU Manufacturing Co, Plympton Street, London NW8 8AB
Olympus OES bronchofibrescope BF10	4865·00	Key Med, Key Med House, Stock Road, Southend on Sea SS2 5QH
Keymed Keylight MS-A Coldlight source	336·00	"

VAT = Value added tax.

The respiratory physician in a Third World district hospital

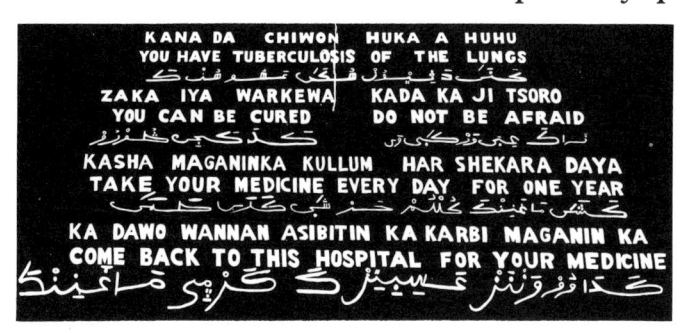

FIG 1—Advice for patients with tuberculosis displayed prominently on wall of the tuberculosis clinic in Zaria, Nigeria.

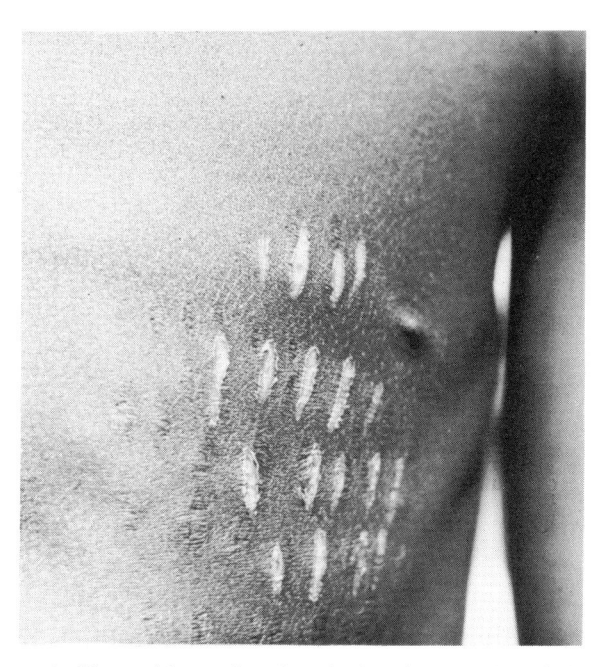

FIG 2—The age of the scars from the native doctor's cuts may be useful in timing the duration of the illness. This man with pleurisy has fresh cuts only a few days old, but older, healed scars suggest a similar illness in the past.

weighing is one of the best ways to assess response to treatment, and a set of scales should be kept in the clinic. Compliance may be checked by looking at the colour of the urine if the patient is taking rifampicin; testing for other drugs is more complicated and needs to be done in a laboratory.[9] In some areas rifampicin commands high prices on the black market for the treatment of gonorrhoea and other conditions—this may be a problem when patients are given several weeks' supply at one time.

Asthma

Asthma is the major non-infectious respiratory problem. The history is crucial in making the diagnosis, and education of the patients is most important in the management of the condition. It may well be worth setting up an asthma clinic. A special nurse(s) or interpreter may be trained to take reliable respiratory histories and to provide explanations and advice to the patients. A duplicated standardised questionnaire using local terminology is useful. The symptoms of chronic asthma may be mistaken for tuberculosis by patients and their relatives, so careful but simple explanations will be needed. The clinic may be a good way to follow up patients with other non-infectious respiratory problems—for example, alveolitis or pulmonary shadowing of unknown cause.

Complicated equipment to test lung function is not required, but a peak flow meter is essential for both diagnosis and management of asthma (fig 3). The best buy is the robust and accurate Wright peak flow meter. Plastic mouthpieces are better than disposable cardboard ones because they may be cleaned and reused. Ideally, each medical ward should have at least one peak flow meter and there should be one in the outpatient area. The Wright mini peak flow meter is an alternative, and is lightweight, strong, washable, and cheaper than the Wright peak flow meter. Bronchodilator pressurised aerosols should be kept in the clinic to assess reversibility of airways obstruction.

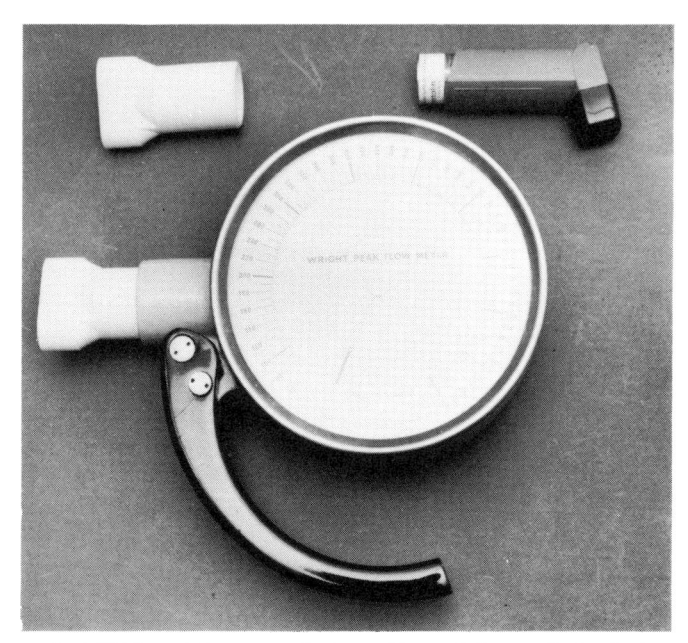

FIG 3—A Wright peak flow meter, plastic reusable mouthpieces, and a β_2 stimulant pressurised inhaler are essential for managing asthma.

It is useful but not essential to have a spirometer to measure simple lung volumes—for example, forced expiratory volume in one second and vital capacity. These measurements help in the diagnosis and monitoring of restrictive and obstructive forms of lung disease. Although expensive and cumbersome, the Vitalograph dry spirometer model R is very satisfactory. Special paper charts are needed, but with care many recordings can be made on each chart. Predicted values for lung function results vary for different ethnic populations, and guidance may be obtained from standard sources of references.[11]

Carrying out skin prick tests may add interest to patient investigations but rarely influences management. Hyposensitisation or avoidance of allergens is usually impracticable. Patterns of positive prick tests have been reported from many developing countries and published in *Clinical Allergy* (Blackwell Scientific Publications). If no published information can be found for a particular area a simple collection of prick test solutions could include glycerosaline control, house dust, *Dermatophagoides farinae* or *Dermatophagoides pteronyssinus*, grass pollen, mixed animal hairs, cockroach, mixed threshings, ascaris, and *Aspergillus fumigatus*. These may be obtained from Bencard or Dome/Hollister-Stier. Solutions have a shelf life of two years at 4°C. Blood lancets, cleaned between use, may be used for pricking the skin.

TREATMENT

The treatment of asthma will depend on the local availability of drugs and their price. Ideally, β_2 stimulant bronchodilators and prophylactic treatment such as steroids or sodium cromoglycate should be given through pressurised inhalers[12]—unfortunately, such treatment is often expensive and scarce. Patients will need repeated instruction on how, when, and why to use the different inhalers. If inhaled prophylactic treatment is not available long term management of asthma is difficult and will depend on the use of oral

The respiratory physician in a Third World district hospital

bronchodilators and the judicious use of oral steroids. Although short courses of steroids are safe, long courses carry appreciable risks in tropical climates.[13]

If possible the management of severe acute asthma should be standardised and displayed on wall charts in the outpatient area and medical wards. Remember that intravenous steroids are expensive and that oral steroids are cheap and work almost as quickly. Although intravenous aminophylline is a cheap and readily available bronchodilator, intermittent nebulised β_2 stimulants (for example, salbutamol, terbutaline) are safer and as effective. If solutions of bronchodilator are available at an affordable price they may be given through a nebuliser chamber driven by an oxygen or air cylinder at a flow rate of 8 l/min. Chambers such as the Intersurgical nebuliser are cheap but robust enough for several uses after cleaning. If oxygen and air cylinders are unavailable, consider buying one or two electric nebuliser compressors such as the heavy duty Aerolyser CFIR or the more fragile Porta-Neb 50 Multivolt that may be operated off a 12 volt DC source. A useful discussion of the problem of managing asthma in the tropics is given elsewhere.[13]

The diagnosis of respiratory failure will be clinical as measurement of arterial blood gas tensions will almost certainly be unavailable. Assisted ventilation for anything apart from a very short time is impracticable in most medical wards in Third World district hospitals because of difficulties in supervising the patient and obtaining (and maintaining) suitable equipment.

Pleural disease

To investigate the cause of pleural effusions by pleural aspiration a large glass syringe, three way tap, and needles for aspiration together with Abrams pleural biopsy needles are needed. A modified version of the Abrams instrument has a three way tap attached. Pleural biopsy specimens should be sent for culture for tuberculosis as well as histological examination. Intercostal drainage of pneumothoraces, effusions, and empyemas requires a selection of Malecot red rubber intercostal drains, an introducer, trocar, and cannula, and a simple underwater drainage system. It is useful but not essential to have at least one cheap and sturdy Roberts low volume electric suction pump for stubborn pneumothoraces and to ensure that the pleural fluid is removed completely. Simple pneumothoraces and empyemas may be managed by repeated needle aspiration in the outpatient department.[14]

Bronchoscopy

A fibreoptic chronoscope is indispensible for respiratory physicians in developed countries, where its major use is in the diagnosis of lung cancer. In this respect its use is limited in the Third World because lung cancer is less common and when it is diagnosed effective treatment is seldom available. Furthermore, fibreoptic bronchoscopes and the accessory equipment are expensive and easily damaged and require specialist servicing. Nevertheless, thought should be given to buying a fibreoptic bronchoscope so that an endoscopy referral centre may be set up to serve several local hospitals. This centre should, in turn, link up to a thoracic surgical centre. If your hospital already has a gastrointestinal fibreoptic endoscopy service it is important to ensure that all endoscopes and equipment are from one manufacturer who can provide good local service facilities. The new range of Olympus endoscopes have the advantage that the whole endoscope is resistant to water and may be totally immersed in sterilising fluid without damage. The Olympus OES bronchofibrescope model BF-10 together with the basic Keymed MS-A cold light source is a good general purpose system. A suction machine will be required.

Although a fibreoptic bronchoscope is not essential, bronchoscopy is required from time to time in all district hospitals to look for foreign bodies, investigate large haemoptyses, manage patients with chest injuries, and aspirate retained secretions and plugs of sputum. In one hospital in Kuwait 250 aspirated foreign bodies were removed over 14 years (about three quarters of these were melon seeds).[15] A set of rigid metal bronchoscopes—paediatric, small adult, and large adult sizes—together with a light source and a simple Venturi jet ventilation system are necessary to undertake this investigation.

Additional points

It is essential to have ready access to the radiology department in the hospital. Complicated apparatus and developing are not needed: good quality posteroanterior and lateral chest radiographs will suffice in most cases. Tomography is rarely required. Bronchography needs no extra equipment except aqueous Dionosil contrast medium, a soft rubber catheter, and a local anaesthetic solution.

Respiratory problems related to work may well be encountered if there are local industries with inadequate safeguards to health. Even traditional crafts may be associated with pneumoconiosis—for example, grindstone cutting is associated with silicosis in northern Nigeria.[16] Diagnosis will depend on taking a good respiratory history from the patient and a knowledge of the industrial process concerned.[17] A small supply of standard mini Wright peak flow meters is useful for self monitoring at work and at home if work related asthma is identified as a local problem.

The importance of teaching special nurses and interpreters has already been mentioned, but the education process must be wider. Every effort should be made to set up lectures and discussion groups for doctors, nurses, and other paramedical staff (physiotherapists, health visitors, village dispensers, etc) to teach them about the common medical and respiratory conditions and their modern management.

Preventive medicine will have a major impact on the community's health, and the respiratory physician should play an active part in, for example, promoting and organising BCG vaccination and campaigning against smoking and cigarette advertising. The latter is particularly important otherwise smoking related disease will become as common in developing countries as it is in the West.

I am grateful for the advice that I obtained in preparing this article from Dr J Cookson, Dr S Fisher, Dr B Harrison and Dr R Wolstenholme, all of whom have also practised respiratory medicine abroad. My thanks also to my wife for typing the drafts and the manuscript.

References

1 Shaper AG, Shaper L. Analysis of medical admission to Mulago hospital, 1957. *East Afr Med J* 1958;35:647-78.
2 Lawless J, Lawless MM, Garden AS. Admission and mortality in a children's ward in an urban tropical hospital. *Lancet* 1966;ii:1175-6.
3 Woolcock AJ, Blackburn CRB. Chronic lung disease in the territory of Papua New Guinea—an epidemiological study. *Australasian Annals of Medicine* 1967;16:11-9.
4 Wolstenholme RJ. Bronchial asthma in the southern Maldives. *Clin Allergy* 1979;9:325-32.
5 Aderele WI. Bronchial asthma in Nigerian children. *Arch Dis Child* 1979;54:448-53.
6 Macfarlane JT, Adegboye DS, Warrell MJ. Mycoplasma pneumoniae and the aetiology of lobar pneumonia in northern Nigeria. *Thorax* 1979;34:713-9.
7 Warrell DA. Respiratory tract infections in the tropics. *Practitioner* 1975;215:740-6.
8 King M. *Medical care in developing countries*. London: Oxford University Press, 1967.
9 Ross JD, Horne NW. *Modern drug treatment in tuberculosis*. 6th ed. London: Chest, Heart and Stroke Association, 1983.
10 Crofton J, Douglas A. *Respiratory diseases*. 3rd ed. Oxford: Blackwell Scientific Publications, 1981.
11 Cotes JE. *Lung function*. 4th ed. Oxford: Blackwell Scientific Publications, 1979.
12 Clark TJH, Godfrey S. *Asthma*. 2nd ed. London: Chapman and Hall, 1983.
13 Warrell DA, Fawcett IW, Harrison BDW, et al. Bronchial asthma in the Nigerian savanna region. *Q J Med* 1975;174:325-47.
14 Riordan JF. Management of spontaneous pneumothorax. *Br Med J* 1984;289:71.
15 Abdulmajid OA, Ebeid AM, Motaweh MM, Kleibo IS. Aspirated foreign bodies in the tracheobronchial tree—report of 250 cases. *Thorax* 1976;31:635-40.
16 Warrell DA, Harrison BDW, Fawcett IW, et al. Silicosis among grindstone cutters in the north of Nigeria. *Thorax* 1975;30:389-98.
17 Parkes WR. *Occupational lung disorders*. 2nd ed. London: Butterworths, 1982.

ORTHOPAEDIC AIDS AT LOW COST

KO DE RUŸTER, OTTO LELIEVELD

Western orthopaedic aids are seldom suitable for Third World countries. They are often made from costly materials and require complex technology for their manufacture. In countries where resources are limited alternative aids must be made, and here we describe some of the aids and techniques that are in use in the physiotherapy department of a district hospital, leprosarium, and school for the handicapped in Zambia.

Orthopaedic aids need to be simple and durable, and in our view it is important that items are made locally, using raw materials and skills that are readily available. This obviates the problem of having to get foreign currency (which is difficult) to import the items of equipment. Home produced aids are also less expensive and easy to repair, and their production creates local employment.

Crutches and walking aids

We make four types of crutches, three of wood and one of metal. The axilla crutch is made of wood, with a piece of car tyre at the bottom for protection. The top is made of cotton wool, foam, or another soft material and covered with leather (fig 1(a)). This type of crutch is suitable for small children. The two other types of axilla crutch shown in figure 1 have a better handgrip and are suitable for adults. Elbow crutches may also be made out of metal rods with a piece of rubber tubing to pad the handgrip (fig 1(d)). Welding equipment is needed to make this sort of crutch, but it has the advantage of being stronger than the wooden crutch and avoids putting pressure on the axilla. If welding equipment is available other items—for example, walking aids (fig 1(e)) and adjustable parallel bars—may be made. (Fixed parallel bars may also be made of bamboo and various other woods.)

Simple prosthetic above and below knee walking aids may be made out of plaster of Paris, wood, and metal strips (fig 2). Extra layers of plaster of Paris are used to connect the metal strips on to the plaster case. The kneeling prosthesis is attached to the leg by leather straps.

Sandals

Thick soled sandals are needed to protect the feet of patients with leprosy who have lost normal sensation. Different types of shoe may be made to suit the individual, but they are all designed to prevent damage from sharp stones and to provide a soft top layer to prevent pressure sores developing. The materials that we use include:

(1) used car tyres for a firm sole,
(2) tropical or microcellular rubber as a soft protective insole,
(3) leather straps (or straps made of the inner tube of a car),

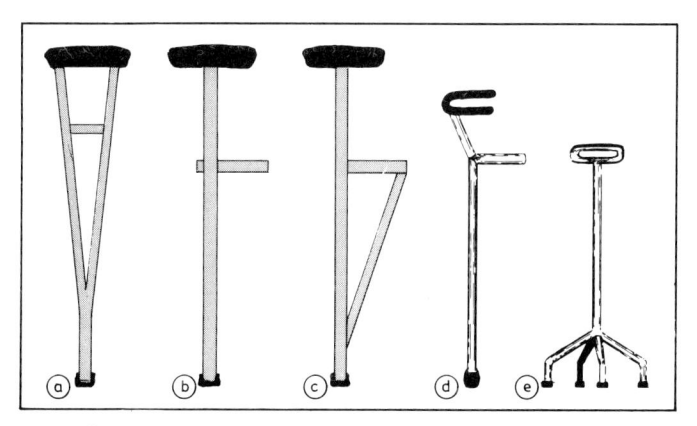

FIG 1—Crutches and walking aids.

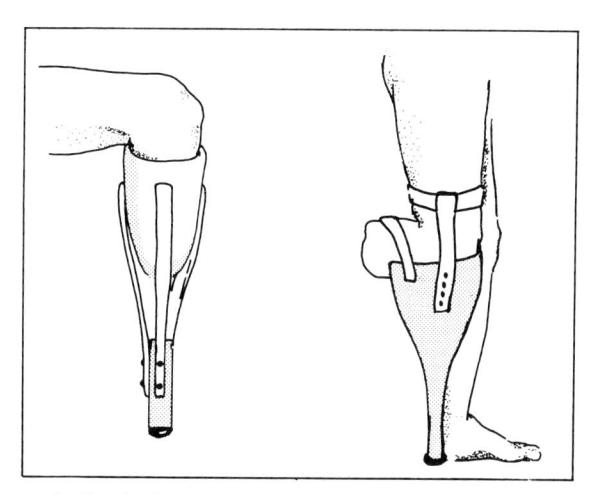

FIG 2—Prosthetic walking aids.

(4) buckles and rivets (when rivets are not available the buckles may be stitched on),
(5) glue,
(6) nylon or cotton threads to stitch the straps on to the tyre.

The sandals are made as shown in figure 3. In brief, the patient puts his foot on a tropical or microcellular rubber sheet and the foot size is drawn and cut out. Leather straps are passed through slits cut in the microcellular rubber and stitched on firmly. The sole of microcellular rubber is then glued on to a broad piece of car tyre, and once the glue is dry the shape of the sandal is cut out of the tyre. Patients with normally shaped feet can usually be fitted from a stock of standard shoes of varying sizes,

Orthopaedic aids at low cost

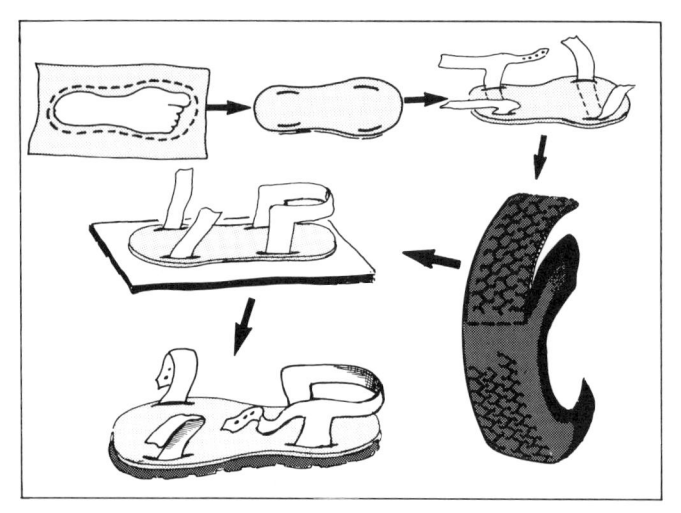

FIG 3—Simply made sandals.

but for those who have lost toes or have other deformities each shoe must be custom made to ensure a good fit. (Nails should never be used for they may cause pressure sores.) This type of sandal is very cheap to produce and usually lasts for about a year.

Calipers

Above and below knee calipers are used to control movement of the leg. They may be adapted to prevent motion, to limit joint motion to the normal range or a portion of the normal range, to correct or prevent the development of deformity, and, finally, to compensate for muscle weakness. We have found that splints and calipers are especially useful in treating patients with acute poliomyelitis, postpolio paralysis, cerebral palsy, and various orthopaedic conditions such as clubfoot and knock knees. The above knee caliper (fig 4) may be made with simple materials and tools and is cheap, strong, and easy to repair. It is based on the caliper that was designed by Dr Huckstep in Uganda in the 1960s.

Production of a below knee caliper is similar to that of an above knee caliper, the only difference being that the ring is horizontal under the knee. Both types of caliper should be moulded around the ankle if the patient has a fixed varus or valgus deformity. A piece of leather placed anteriorly on the knee is used to keep the knee in 0° of extension or in as much extension as is possible. Two square pieces of leather are cut in sizes ranging from 6×6 cm to 13×13 cm and sewn together. One piece is cut from soft leather and the second from stronger leather with a round hole cut in the middle to prevent too much pressure on the patella. A posterior knee leather is used to support an unstable knee and is useful in genu recurvatum. The knee is put in 0° of extension when the caliper is applied and measurements are then taken. The strap should be 5-7 cm broad. With the same materials a knock knee strap may be made to prevent or correct a valgus deformity of the knee. A square piece of leather, about

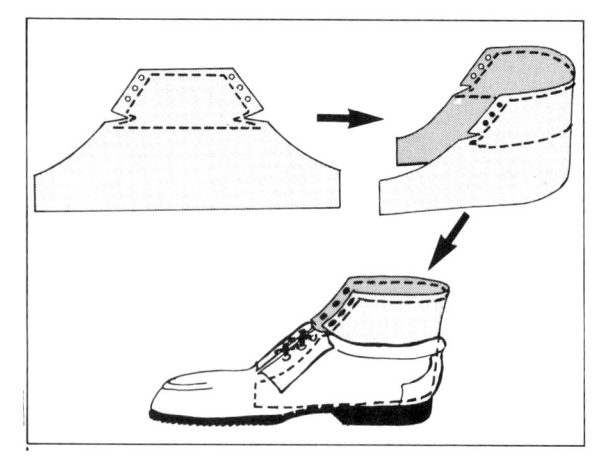

FIG 5—Additional shoe support.

10×10 cm, is used with two straps on top with a buckle on one side. This side of the strap should be long enough to avoid pressure on the skin. An ankle T strap, placed laterally or medially, may be used to prevent or correct a varus or valgus position of the ankle. Finally, a leather ankle strap is necessary to hold both ends of the caliper into the shoe.

A caliper may be fitted into a normal shoe with a rubber heel by drilling two holes in the sides of the heel of the shoe. If the patient cannot afford a shoe a clog is made out of wood with some

An exact contour of the leg is drawn on a large piece of paper. Measurements are taken and added to the plan

The caliper is made from a round steel bar, with a reinforcement rod 6-10 mm diameter depending on age and weight of the patient.

The ring of the caliper is padded with soft material and then covered with leather

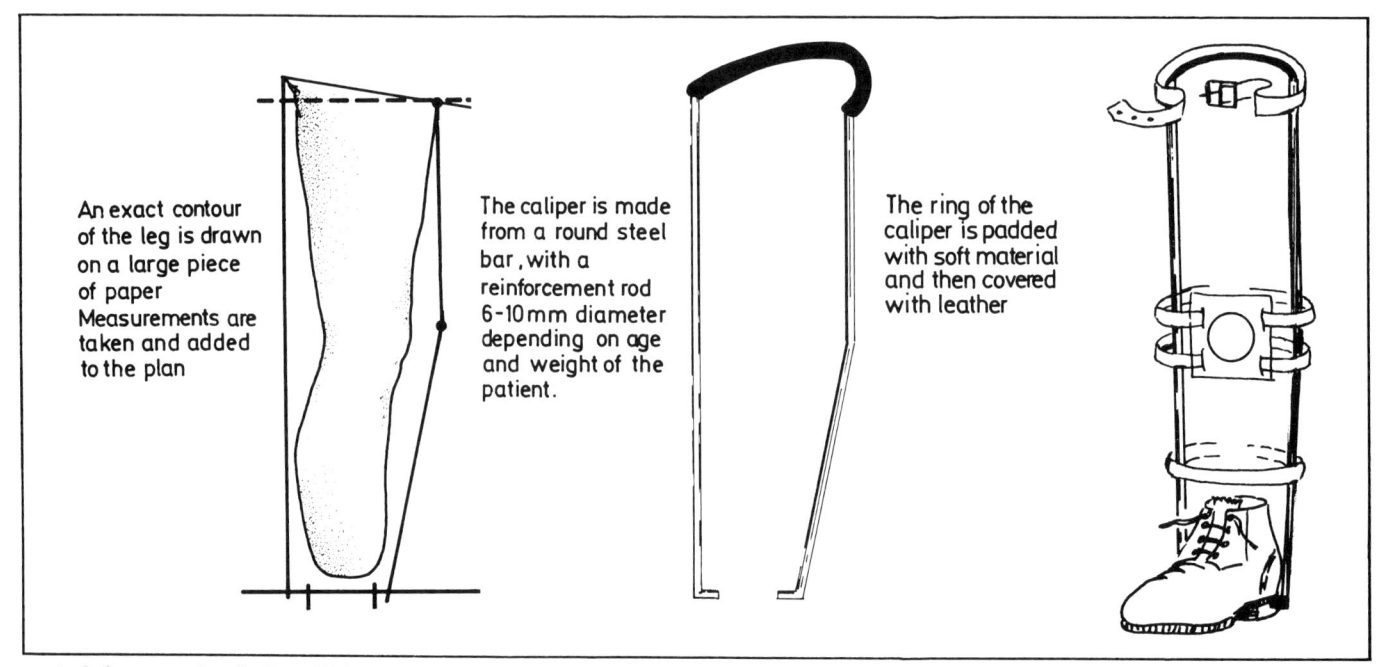

FIG 4—Left, construction of calipers. Right, assembled caliper showing knee piece and attachment to shoe.

Orthopaedic aids at low cost

leather strappings on top. Sometimes a normal shoe does not give enough support and it will be necessary to adapt the shoe into a boot. This may be done by cutting out a piece of leather and stitching it on to the shoe (fig 5). A drop foot may be controlled by a back check stop: a metal pipe in front of a bar is bent and flattened at the ends, which stand vertically. The caliper goes into the pipe, and the ends of the flattened bar permit dorsiflexion but not plantar flexion. Patients with polio may have shortening of the affected legs and need a shoe raise, which may be made out of layers of tropical sheets glued together with a final layer of car tyre.

The items described above have all been made and put to practical use in a district hospital. Furthermore, I have found that these simple, durable aids serve their purpose equally as well as their western counterparts.

Recommended reading

Simple Orthopaedic Aids by Chris Dartnell. This covers how to set up a workshop and gives full details and simple drawings of the production of orthopaedic aids using simple materials. It is available from the Leonard Cheshire Foundation International, Leonard Cheshire House, 26-29 Maunsel Street, London SW1P 2QN, price £2·50 plus p and p.

Poliomyelitis, a guide for developing countries including appliances and rehabilitation for the disabled by Dr Huckstep. London: Churchill Livingstone.

Footwear manual on leprosy. Available from the London leprosy mission (contact Jean Watson).

OPHTHALMOLOGY IN DEVELOPING COUNTRIES

JOHN SANDFORD-SMITH

In the West ophthalmology is sometimes considered to be a minor specialty, but in developing countries it is one of the most important because the prevalence of blindness in many rural areas ranges from 1 to even 5%, compared with about 0·1% in most Western countries. Ophthalmological disorders represent not only a larger problem but also a different one: in developed countries the most common cause of blindness is degenerative or vascular disorders of the retina while in the developing countries five major diseases are responsible for most of the blindness—namely, trachoma, xerophthalmia, cataract, onchocerciasis, and glaucoma.

Major causes of blindness

Trachoma is common throughout the tropics but especially where there is a combination of unhygienic living conditions, a dry dusty atmosphere, and flies. At least two million people are blinded by this disorder, and it causes discomfort and partial visual loss in about another hundred million.[1] The trachoma organism is spread from eye to eye, usually in young children, by close contact and particularly by flies. Trachoma may be a recurrent disease because one attack confers only a low level of immunity. Recurrent episodes cause increasingly severe conjunctival scarring. Poor hygiene also predisposes towards a high incidence of other types of conjunctivitis, especially adenovirus and bacterial conjunctivitis, which further increase the severity of the conjunctival and corneal scarring. The most effective preventive measure is to promote good hygiene to decrease the fly population and lessen the risk of direct eye to eye spread by contact in young children. Intermittent use of tetracycline eye ointment is also helpful both for treatment and to control the spread of the disease in the community by cutting down the number of active carriers. Tetracycline ointment twice daily for five days each month for six months is the schedule recommended by the World Health Organisation.[2]

Nutritional corneal ulceration is one of the most distressing causes of blindness because it affects primarily young and underprivileged children. In Asia alone it afflicts at least one hundred thousand children each year.[3] The causes are complex—the most important are a dietary deficiency of vitamin A and measles. Vitamin A intake may be increased by nutritional advice, by fortification of foods, or by giving capsules of vitamin A every six months. Measles may be prevented by vaccination.

Cataract occurs in all communities but is thought to develop at a younger age in hot countries. About three million people in Africa and five million people in India are blind as a result of cataracts.[1] Of the five major causes of blindness, this is the only one that is treatable. Prevention is at present impossible, but simple eye surgery should restore useful sight.

Onchocerciasis or river blindness due to the *Onchocerca volvulus* worm is found in the Savannah region of central Africa, with pockets of infection in central America and Yemen. In many villages its effects are devastating. Blindness usually develops between the ages of 20 and 40. Prevention may be achieved by controlling the insect vector, and the World Health Organisation (working in the Volta river basin in West Africa) is using insecticide spray to control the similium fly larvae, which are found in small fast flowing streams and rivers. It plans to keep this up for about 20 years because that is the estimated life cycle of the worm. Clinical trials are being carried out on several new drugs which may be effective against the parasitic worm and its larvae. The most promising drug is ivermectin.

Glaucoma occurs in all communities and is an increasingly important cause of blindness with advancing age. Acute glaucoma is rare in negroes, but they are more susceptible to chronic glaucoma. The only realistic way of detecting early glaucoma that I can think of is to have facilities for eye examination and tonometry available throughout the community. This is obviously a counsel of perfection, but wherever appropriately trained primary health care workers or ophthalmic nurses are active in the community they should be able to increase the detection of primary glaucoma in its early stages.

Problems in practising prevention of blindness

Another important feature of ophthalmology in developing countries is the variety of eye disease in different areas. Variations in climate, insect vectors, social surroundings, and nutrition profoundly affect the pattern of eye disease. For example, in Africa on the edge of the Sahara Desert dust, glare, and flies are associated with a high incidence of blindness from trachoma, and corneal conditions such as pterygium and solar keratopathy. Further south in the Savannah dust and flies become less of a problem and the incidence of trachoma falls. This, however, is the zone for onchocerciasis, which in some areas may devastate the entire community. Further south still, in the tropical rain forest, diseases like that due to *Loa-loa*, which causes acute oedema of the eyelid, and nutritional optic atrophy from cassava are found. Throughout Africa there is a high incidence of measles, corneal ulcers, vernal conjunctivis (chronic allergic conjunctivitis), and leprosy affecting the eye.

To confront this vast and varied problem of eye disease with limited resources and a shortage of skilled staff, not only different technology but a different philosophy of what ophthalmology is all about is needed. Western ophthalmology is mainly concerned with curative treatment, and the equipment used in diagnosis and surgical treatment is complex and expensive. In developing countries prevention is all important, and although Western postgraduate training and degrees are highly valued, such training is not suited to tackling the major blinding diseases in rural communities. Most doctors who have obtained their ophthalmological training in the West go into clinical practice in the big cities and have little contact with the poor rural areas. The people who live there (who make up most of the blind people) are, therefore, poorly served, and for most their only

Ophthalmology in developing countries

There are encouraging signs that a more community oriented type of ophthalmic care is being provided in some countries—for example, the mobile eye hospitals, eye camps, and eye safaris in the Indian subcontinent and in some parts of Africa. These are sponsored by the government or by voluntary agencies and offer specialist eye care to the rural communities. The type of service that they usually offer is screening all the local population who complain of problems with their eyes. Those who need medical treatment or glasses are, whenever possible, given them, and those who need simple surgery —for example, for correction of trachomatous entropion, glaucoma, or removal of cataracts—may have that surgery performed locally. Cataracts may be removed very cheaply by a small surgical team: usually a nurse prepares the patient and gives a local anaesthetic, cleans the face and eye, and applies sterile drapes. Ideally, the surgical team has more than one operating table and the surgeon can go from table to table doing simple cataract extractions. This entails making a limbal incision in the eye, a broad iridectomy, removal of the lens, and putting in three or four corneal scleral sutures. In this way a team of two doctors, six to eight nurses, and various unskilled orderlies may get through 100 operations a day. A patient may have his cataract removed (including the price of the drugs and dressings) and be given a pair of spectacles to restore his vision to normal for about US$10 (fig 3).

More complex surgical problems—for example, retinal detachments and corneal grafting—are not usually carried out under such circumstances. In some cases the mobile eye clinic provides only a diagnostic service and medical treatment. Patients who need surgery are identified and sent elsewhere.

Equipment

Snellen's chart for testing visual acuity and a pin hole test that distinguishes refractive errors from eye diseases are essential. A black screen for testing visual fields is helpful, but a simple confrontation test using one's own fingers will detect serious field defects.

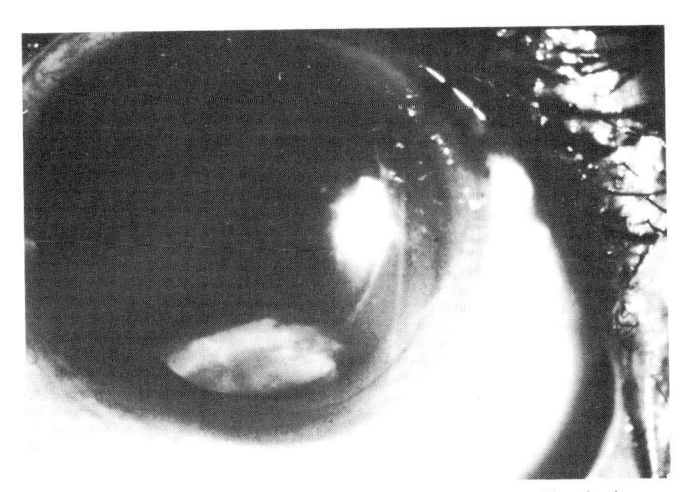

FIG 1—An eye after couching for cataract. Itinerant couchers are still active in some parts of the world. A needle is inserted at the limbus and the lens pushed into the vitreous. The opaque lens can just be seen, through the dilated pupil lying in the lower half of the vitreous. Unfortunately blindness from uveitis or endophthalmitis is the usual result.

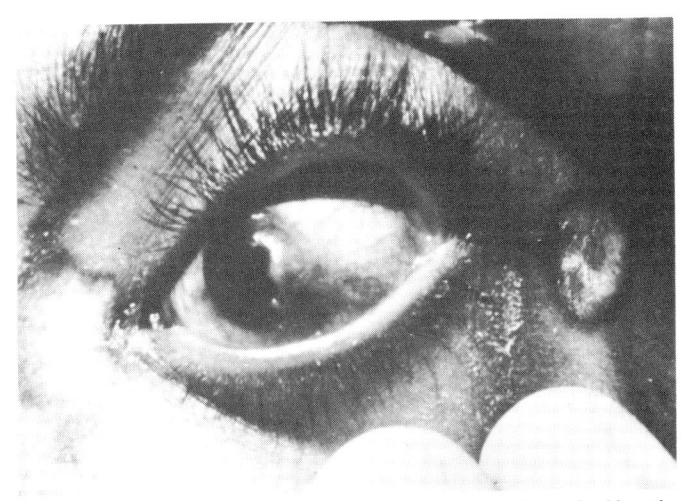

FIG 2—A patient with vernal conjunctivitis. Cautery has been applied to the skin at the inner and outer canthus.

treatment is from unqualified, traditional healers. Although the World Health Organisation is encouraging cooperation with traditional healers in many branches of medicine, this is not advisable in ophthalmology, for unskilled interference is of limited value and may be disastrous (figs 1, 2).

What, then, is needed to provide an adequate ophthalmic service in the Third World? Not lots of money, not lots of equipment, not even lots of specialists packed like sardines in the middle class areas of the big cities, but a service that is oriented towards the rural areas and prevention. This may be achieved with limited resources and equipment, provided that it is realistically planned and carried out by dedicated workers. There must be good two way contact between the community and the eye specialist. The best way to achieve this is to train primary health care workers or ophthalmic nurses to make the initial contact and then liaise with the ophthalmologist. Village and community leaders may be taught how to prevent blindness from diseases like trachoma, vitamin A deficiency, and measles. Other specialists may be enlisted to help—for example, horticulturists can identify foods rich in vitamin A that may be grown locally. Thus eye specialists must be encouraged to spend some of their time training and supervising medical assistants, nurses, dispensers, and primary health care workers. Obviously most specialists will want a base in a major city, but ophthalmology, with its easily portable equipment, lends itself to mobile work. It is much easier for one ophthalmologist and one trained nurse to travel 200 miles than for a hundred bewildered, blind, and elderly patients with their escorts to travel in the opposite direction.

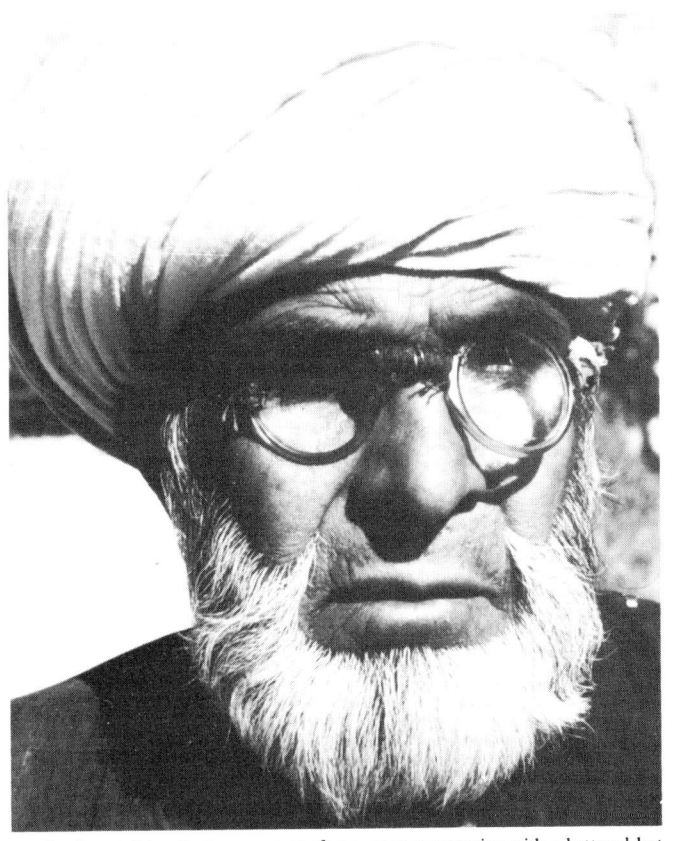

FIG 3—A grateful patient some years after a cataract operation with a battered but functional pair of glasses.

Ophthalmology in developing countries

An ophthalmoscope is essential. Many people do not realise that an ophthalmoscope may also be used to examine the front of the eye as well as the fundus. By holding the instrument as for fundus examination but using a strong positive lens (about +15 or +20) a magnified and illuminated view of the front of the eye is obtained. If the pupil is dilated slight opacities in the cornea, lens, or vitreous may be seen standing out against the red fundus reflex. A simple torch light and magnifying lens are also helpful for examining the cornea and conjunctiva, and fluorescein paper is essential for detecting corneal ulcers. A tonometer for measuring intraocular pressure is another essential item. The old fashioned Schiotz tonometer is cheap, and if kept scrupulously clean and used correctly it is reliable. Applanation tonometers give more consistent results; the Perkins tonometer and the Glaucotest (made in Germany by Heine) are two useful examples.

A simple microscope to examine skin snips for microfilaria is important in areas where onchocerciasis is endemic. More expensive items include a slit lamp and a binocular indirect ophthalmoscope (for example, the Schultz Crock, which has rechargeable batteries, costs £500). These are expensive but provide a superb view of the front and back of the eye respectively and are essential diagnostic tools for the specialist working in a major eye centre.

Surgery

Nearly all surgery on adults may be done under local anaesthetic. Ophthalmic surgical instruments need to be of good quality and should be packed, handled, and sterilised with great care. Some magnification is necessary for most eye surgery, but an operating microscope is an expensive luxury and perfectly adequate magnification for all but the finest procedures may be achieved using a telescopic pair of operating glasses that will magnify from ×2 to ×4. Of these I recommend those made by Zeiss (East Germany), which cost about £80. Most of the instruments described are robust and, provided the batteries are not left to run down and corrode (and instruments are used for which local batteries and a good supply of bulbs are available), there should be no great problem in operating them. Slit lamps may be run off car batteries with appropriate connections if they are used by mobile eye teams.

Cataract surgery is the most common operation, but other important procedures include the correction of trachomatous entropion and the treatment of glaucoma by iridectomy or a drainage operation. Ideally, only a trained specialist should perform eye surgery of any sort, but there is such a shortage of trained ophthalmologists in many developing countries that either a general duties doctor or a nurse with specific ophthalmological training may be taught some of the basic surgical skills. They should then be able to carry out safely the three procedures mentioned above, which encompass up to 90% of the potentially treatable blinding conditions in rural communities.

Drugs

Basic ophthalmology does not require many drugs, and most drops and ointments may be made up by the pharmacist. Tetracycline ointment is the best local treatment for trachoma and chloroamphenicol a good all round antibiotic. Local steroids are effective in the treatment of uveitis and other forms of inflammatory eye disease but may result in serious complications if they are misused. Atropine is the best long acting mydriatic, but a short acting mydriatic—for example, homatropine—should be used to dilate the pupil before examining the fundus. Pilocarpine is needed for patients with glaucoma, to prepare the eye for surgery. Medical treatment of glaucoma is usually inappropriate because the patients cannot afford the drugs and are unlikely to comply with long term regular treatment. Many antibiotics and steroid preparations may be injected subconjunctivally to treat severe infection or inflammation of the eye. Gentamicin is particularly useful as a broad spectrum injectable antibiotic for bacterial corneal ulcers or endophthalmitis. A supply of placebo drops (zinc sulphate or saline) is useful in some countries where the prevailing opinion is that "a doctor who doesn't prescribe any medicine can't be any good."

Spectacles

In developing countries facilities for manufacturing and fitting spectacles vary widely but spectacles can usually be manufactured locally. Two main types of glasses are needed: spectacles for near vision for elderly presbyopic patients with a power of about +2·5 diopters and aphakic glasses for patients who have had cataracts removed, with a power of about +10 diopters (fig 3).

In conclusion, the ophthalmic services in common with other medical services in the Third World are often inadequate. The unique challenge of ophthalmology is that most blindness is avoidable without enormous expenditure. The obstacles to prevention are mostly human—unwillingness to work and travel in rural areas, fear of teaching surgical skills to non-specialists, and uninterest in community health and preventive medicine—and these must be overcome.

The Institute of Ophthalmology in London holds a six month course on the prevention of blindness in developing countries. The course is organised for doctors, nurses, and administrators and is particularly concerned to teach the very varied skills needed to provide comprehensive eye care.

References

1 International Agency for the Prevention of Blindness, ed. *World blindness and its prevention.* Oxford: Oxford University Press, 1980.
2 World Health Organisation. *Guide to trachoma control.* Geneva: WHO, 1981.
3 World Health Organisation. *Vitamin A deficiency and xerophthalmia.* Geneva: WHO, 1976.

Further reading

Jones BR. The prevention of blindness from trachomas. *Transactions of the Ophthalmological Society of the UK* 1974;95:16-33.
Somer A. *Field guide to the detection and contact of xerophthalmia.* Geneva: WHO, 1978.
Anderson J, Fuglsang H. Ocular onchocerciasis. *Trop Dis Bull* 1977;74:4.
World Health Organisation. *Symptomology, pathology and diagnosis of onchocerciasis.* Geneva: WHO, 1974.

ESSENTIAL MEDICINES IN THE THIRD WORLD

P F D'ARCY

For many Third World countries health care is only one problem on a priority scale that is dominated by poverty, starvation, refugees, a growing population, political unrest, and corruption. Furthermore, the type of health care problems in Third World countries is quite different from that in industrialised countries (fig 1), and infectious diseases remain a problem. Despite this high incidence of infectious diseases such countries have only a small share in the total world use of medicines (fig 2).[1] In the least developed countries spending on drugs per person per year comes to less than US$1, whereas in the industrialised countries the corresponding figure is $70 or more.[2] In many countries this is because imported drugs are too expensive and there are no facilities for the local manufacture of drugs.

If health care is to be given a priority in developing countries, treatment and medication must be available to the sick patient at the time of need. It is a stark fact, however, that throughout most of the Third World almost three quarters of the population has no access to basic health services. Hospitals and clinics are grouped in the major urban areas while most people live in the rural areas and are more or less neglected. Therefore most patients present at hospitals and clinics late, when their disease is advanced. Lack of transport, poor communications, long distances, and a lack of local medical care may transform simple and curable diseases into chronic, crippling, or life threatening conditions. Drawing up a more equitable health care system, based on the development of primary health care, calls for a firm policy on essential drugs to satisfy the real needs of most of the community. Such a policy is lacking in many countries, and even if patients reach their district hospital the drugs required for their treatment may not be available.

Availability of medicines

In this article I propose to question why "not available" is the most common answer to a request for even simple medicines, and why so many patients in the Third World are deprived of the benefits of effective treatment. The answer to the question, why not available? is difficult because usually various factors have to be considered and these may include inefficiency and corruption. In my experience common explanations why particular drugs or formulations were not available include:

(1) Because they are too expensive and insufficient funds are available to maintain a constant supply.

(2) Because they are in the central store but transport is not available to distribute them to clinics and hospitals.

(3) Because the government has a foreign exchange problem and the annual drug tender has been delayed.

(4) Because they are held up at the railway station, docks, airport, etc.

(5) Because they have been lost (pilfered) in transit.

(6) Because the papers (import documents, customs clearance certificates, etc) have been lost.

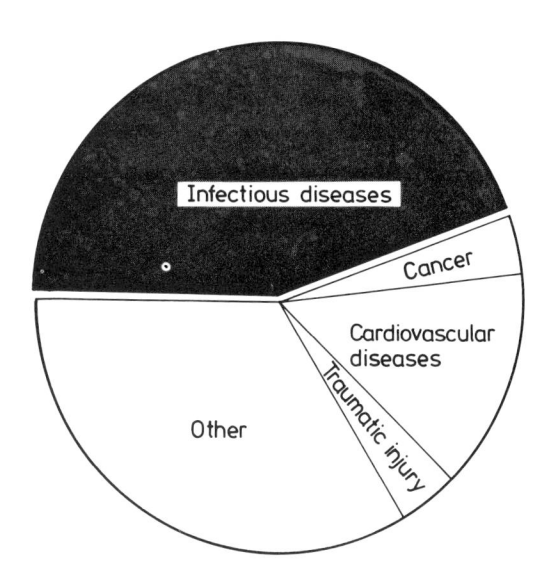

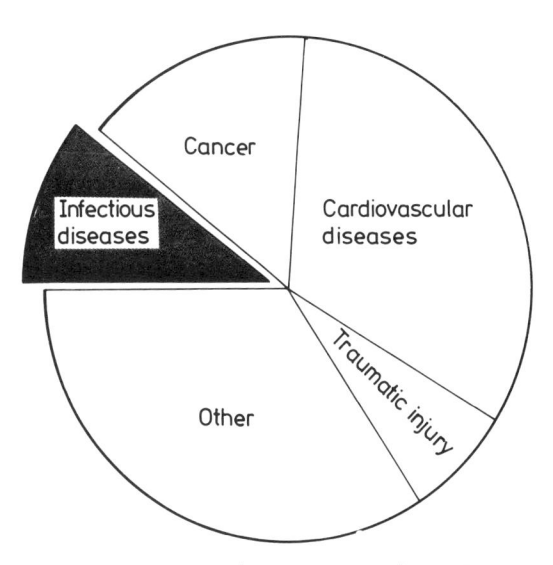

FIG 1—Deaths by cause in the rich and poor countries (modified from Taylor[1]).

(7) Because they have deteriorated in the central drug store (heat, damp, etc).

(8) Because the replacement supply was not ordered in time. The list continues ad infinitum.

Essential medicines in the Third World

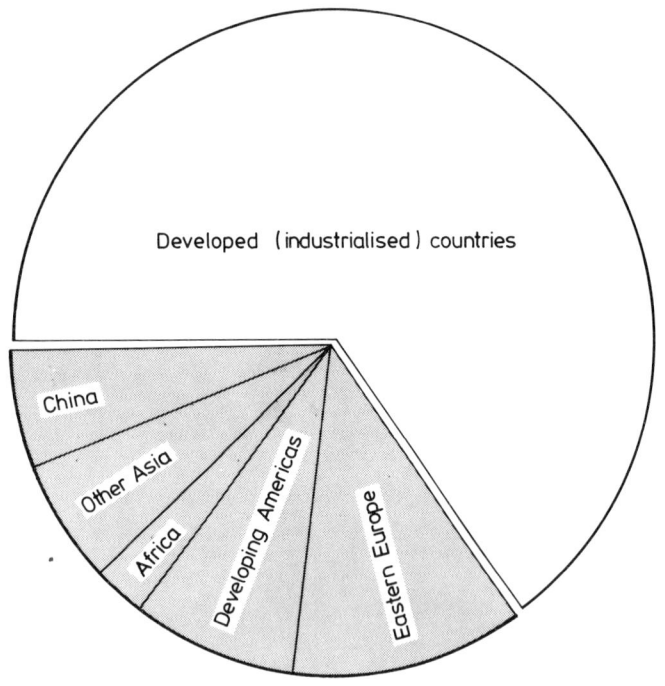

FIG 2—World pharmaceutical consumption; total US$76 000m in 1980—manufacturers' prices (modified from Taylor[1]).

Essential drugs

What, therefore, is the solution? First and foremost, the ministry of health in the developing country needs to integrate a programme of importation of drugs (or their local manufacture if possible) within a coherent policy on primary health care. This requires political stability because such programmes must be long term; it also assumes that health care budgets are given adequate priority. Importation of drugs should be through a regular drug tender, and substantial saving may be achieved by purchasing generic preparations rather than branded or proprietary products. The move among some major pharmaceutical companies to manufacture generic products is particularly welcome, because it increases their availability and allays anxiety about their quality.

Selection of drugs should be based on the model list of essential drugs of the World Health Organisation (WHO),[3] which may be modified or augmented according to the specific needs of the country. Whenever possible, priority should be given in the drug tender to locally based pharmaceutical industries, which should be encouraged to manufacture formulations based on the list of essential drugs. The responsibility for quality control should rest with a government laboratory which can ensure that preparations manufactured locally and imported products or raw materials are of a satisfactory standard. Setting up a quality control laboratory may, however, be difficult in small countries which lack the necessary financial, physical, and trained resources, and with these countries in mind the WHO drug certification scheme has been introduced to ensure that imported drugs conform to international standards. Use of this scheme might be combined with more efficient use of the quality control laboratories that are already established, some of which have been set up on a cooperative regional or subregional basis.

Offers of help

Information and guidance on the procedures concerned in obtaining drugs are given by the International Federation of Pharmaceutical Manufacturers Associations (IFPMA). This organisation covers both the developed and the developing world, and its member associations include not only the 100 or so international, research based pharmaceutical companies but also many thousands of small national manufacturing companies producing standard products.[4,5]

The International Federation has taken an active interest in the WHO action programme on essential drugs and, through its international code of pharmaceutical marketing practices,[6] it has done much to counteract the claim by some Third World countries that they are the dumping ground for unwanted, obsolete, and poor quality drugs.[7,8] IFPMA also provides, advises, and runs training courses on topics such as the distribution and procurement of drugs. In addition, courses in quality control of drugs are arranged for trainees from government laboratories and inspection services in the Third World.

Many Third World countries claim that they are not supplied with information about indications, contraindications, and side effects of individual drugs. In response to this, the International Federation has offered to supply (free of charge to government health departments) standard compendia listing this sort of information—for example, the *Physician's Desk Reference* (USA), the Association of the British Pharmaceutical Industry's *Data Sheet Compendium* (UK), the *Rote List* (Federal Republic of Germany), and the *Dictionnaire Vidal* (France). The problem remains, however, that owing to bureaucratic inertia or inefficiency the information contained in these compendia is not always passed on by the health ministry to the practitioners who need it.

Local drug manufacture

The United Nations Industrial Development Organisation (UNIDO) is concerned with helping developing countries to industrialise, and the manufacture of pharmaceuticals is one of the industries that they have singled out for special attention. The United Nations Conference on Trade and Development (UNCTAD) has been negotiating an international code of conduct on the transfer of technology and an agreement by which local manufacturers may gain technical know how from the larger international companies. The WHO and the World Bank—or in some cases regional development banks—are already collaborating in several industrial projects. Clearly if a group of countries got together and agreed to have a single commercial production unit for essential drugs this would count as technical cooperation between developing countries and would attract grants and funding, which is one of the priorities within the United Nations system.[9]

Unfortunately, the development of a locally based pharmaceutical industry does not have priority in some Third World countries, simply because the government is more interested in providing employment in more labour intensive industries, with a predominance of unskilled or semi-skilled jobs. The pharmaceutical industry is not labour intensive and depends largely on a small core of local or expatriate skilled staff. Nevertheless, a local pharmaceutical industry is an important contribution to the overall provision of health care and must be recognised as such, although it does not necessarily produce cheap drugs, nor does the manufacture of essential drug preparations tend to attract large profits. Thus the local industry needs to be protected by concessions to facilitate the import of raw materials, containers, and packaging materials. It is reasonable to expect such concessions provided that the companies are manufacturing essential drugs with a view to improving health care and not producing non-essential proprietary preparations or cosmetics.

Storage and distribution

Even if an adequate supply is ensured there may still be problems of storage and distribution, especially if supplies are centralised in a government drug store. Road and rail systems in developing countries are often poor, so that the distribution of consumable items from urban to rural areas suffers. Medicines should, however, be given priority and not regarded as ordinary items of commerce.

Whereas the role of the medical practitioner is traditionally appreciated and understood in all Third World countries (particularly in the governmental administrative service), that of his pharmaceutical counterpart is less well understood. Many countries

Essential medicines in the Third World

fail to understand that expert pharmaceutical advice is essential not only for drug procurement but also for effective storage, distribution, and legislative control. Many countries rely on inadequately trained dispensers to staff hospital pharmacies, on store keepers to control distribution of drugs from central stores, and on doctors or administrators to control their drug tenders. This is wasteful, and it fails to take account of the skill of the pharmacist and the benefits that can accrue from having expert pharmaceutical advice about the ordering, quality testing, storage, distribution, and supply of medicines.

Hospital manufacture

Local manufacture of pharmaceuticals is invariably thought of as a commercial enterprise, but a lot can be done in the hospital pharmacy provided that expert advice and skills together with the necessary equipment are available. The range of equipment required will depend on which preparations are manufactured, but this need not be extensive. Advice on the choice of equipment, and subsequent servicing, may be obtained from the Third World project of the Fédération Internationale Pharmaceutique.[10 11]

Producing a hospital formulary of essential drugs may cut the hospital's total drug bill, and the manufacture of simple solid and liquid oral dosage forms, topical preparations, injection solutions, and sterile eye preparations may not only save money but also ensure that these preparations are readily available and that they can be freshly prepared according to demand. A formulary—for example, one based on the *British National Formulary*—will also do much to standardise treatments and prevent the prescription of unnecessary preparations.

Containers

Suitable containers for dispensed medicines do not exist in many developing countries. Tablets are dispensed in a screw of paper; liquid formulations are filled into Pepsi Cola bottles; sterile eye ointments are spread on to paper and given to the patient as a crude package; sterile eye drops or lotions are put into cans, bottles, tins, or whatever container the patient can buy at the stall at the entrance to the hospital. Thus the Third World urgently needs an inexhaustible supply of simple plastic universal containers that may be sealed and made air and water tight. Clearly, there is little use in dispensing essential medicines if they are spoilt or allowed to deteriorate almost immediately in unsuitable containers. It would be better to allocate a part of the budget for outpatients' drugs to providing cheap and simple containers. At least one manufacturer in each country should be encouraged to produce a standard container for outpatient use. It has been done for yogurt in some Third World countries, so why not for medicines? It may then be possible to write simple instructions (or draw pictorial labels) on the containers so that the patient uses the medicine correctly. It is practically impossible to write instructions on a screw of paper—I know, I've tried.

References

1 Taylor D. *Medicines, health and the poor world*. London: Office of Health Economics, 1982.
2 Fattorusso V. Essential drugs for the Third World. *World Development* 1983;11:177-9.
3 World Health Organisation. The use of essential drugs. Report of a WHO expert committee. *WHO Tech Rep Ser* 1983;685:1-46.
4 Peretz SM. Pharmaceuticals in the Third World: the problem from the suppliers' point of view. *World Development* 1983;11:259-64.
5 Peretz SM. IFPMA's current activities and involvement with UN agencies. In: *Pharmaceuticals in developing countries. Cost-effectiveness of pharmaceuticals.* (11th IFPMA Assembly, Washington, June 1982.) Zurich: International Federation of Pharmaceutical Manufacturers Associations, 1982:71-80.
6 International Federation of Pharmaceutical Manufacturers Associations. Code of pharmaceutical marketing practices (1981). *World Development* 1983;11:313-5.
7 Melrose D. *Bitter pills. Medicines and the Third World poor*. Oxford: Oxfam Public Affairs Unit, 1982.
8 Muller M. *The health of nations. A north-south investigation*. London: Faber and Faber, 1982.
9 Balasubramaniam K. The main lines of cooperation among developing countries in pharmaceuticals. *World Development* 1983;11:281-7.
10 D'Arcy PF. Action programmes: FIP Third World project. *Pharmacy International* 1983;4:157-8.
11 Fédération Internationale Pharmaceutique. Training and communication: means of solving problems in the Third World. *Pharmacy International* 1983;4:306-10.

Contact addresses

International Federation of Pharmaceutical Manufacturers Associations, 67 rue de St Jean, 1201 Geneva, Switzerland.
United Nations Industrial Development Organisation, Vienna International Centre, PO Box 300, A-1400 Vienna, Austria.
United Nations Conference on Trade and Development, Palais des Nations, CH-1211 Geneva 10, Switzerland.
Fédération Internationale Pharmaceutique, Third World Project, Coordinator: Professor P F D'Arcy, Department of Pharmacy, Queen's University of Belfast, Medical Biology Centre, Lisburn Road, Belfast BT9 7BL, Northern Ireland, United Kingdom.

PRINCIPLES OF HEALTH EDUCATION

JOHN HUBLEY

Health education is an essential component of any programme to improve the health of a community, and it has a major role in promoting:

(a) good health practices; for example, sanitation, clean drinking water, good hygiene, breast feeding, infant weaning, and oral rehydration;

(b) the use of preventive services—for example, immunisation, screening, antenatal and child health clinics;

(c) the correct use of medications and the pursuit of rehabilitation regimens—for example, for tuberculosis and leprosy respectively;

(d) the recognition of early symptoms of disease and promoting early referral;

(e) community support for primary health care and government control measures.

Despite the potential benefits of health education, existing schemes are often inadequate and ineffective. In this article I review a range of experiences in the developing world to identify the ingredients for effective and appropriate health education. The key decisions that form the basis for any planning are decisions over *what* the desired change should be, *where* the health education should take place, *who* should carry it out, and *how* it should be done.

What to change

The first step in planning any health education is to decide what the key problems are and what advice should be given. Well meaning attempts to introduce new practices may fail if they are incompatible with local beliefs and practices.[1] Changes advocated by health educators who are based centrally may be unrealistic locally, so a comprehensive strategy of health education both locally and nationally is necessary. Any proposal for a change of practice should:

(a) be simple to put into practice with the existing knowledge and skills in the community;

(b) fit in with existing life style and culture and not conflict with local beliefs;

(c) not require resources of money, materials, and time that are not available locally;

(d) meet a felt need of the community;

(e) be seen by the people to convey real benefits in the short term, not in the distant future.

To achieve success, health education programmes need to be flexible and modify their advice to fit in with people's circumstances—for example, education about nutrition should be based on foods that are available locally, aids for the disabled made from local materials, latrines built with traditional methods. Local taboos are rarely obstacles to implementing health education; indeed, many traditional beliefs are sound and may actually support the health education programme.[3]

If the change that you wish to promote cannot be modified easily to fit in with the local community, it will be hard to promote it. It may be wise to start with a simple change that does fit in and meets an immediate need, and once that has been accomplished—and the benefits are apparent—the good will and trust generated may help in achieving a more difficult objective. Health education depends on continuous dialogue with the community to find acceptable solutions to meet their needs.

Where should health education take place?

A starting point for improving health education is a careful study of existing clinics, health centres, outpatient departments, and hospitals, but every encounter between a health worker and the community is an opportunity and health workers need to allot sufficient time for this (fig 1). They must also be

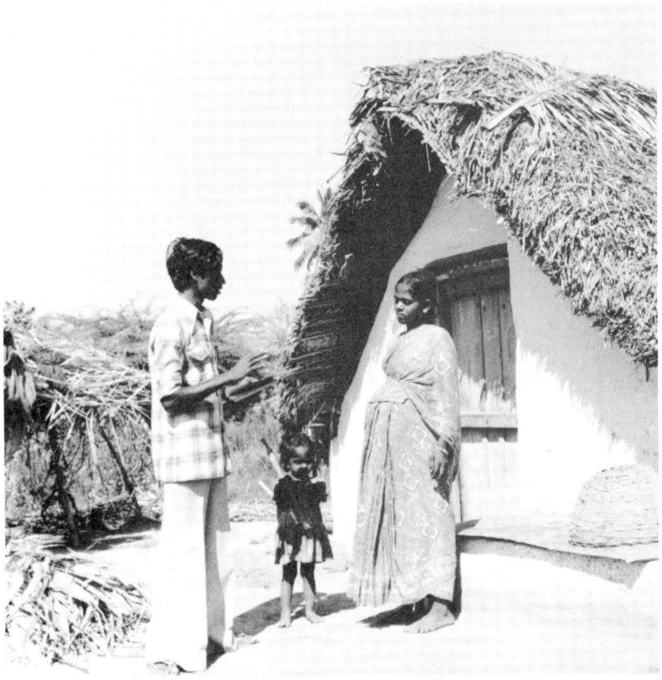

FIG 1—Health education should be taken out into the community: a health care worker contacting a pregnant woman at home as part of a rural health programme in Tamil Nadu, South India.

encouraged to make full use of the surroundings and waiting areas for displays and demonstrations. Quiet areas where talks and small group discussions can be held are valuable, and it is important to remember that the most powerful way to implement change is to show that the staff themselves practise the preventive measures that they are recommending to the community.

Home visits and follow up are essential parts of any community based health education project, so the workload and schedules of duty of health workers need to be organised to allow them sufficient time for these activities. Opportunities for health education may be provided in those places where people come together—for example, in shops, market places,[4] community centres, churches, and so on. Health workers may also join forces with others to set up groups—for example, mothers' clubs, youth groups, and preschool crèches. Such groups fulfil a social need as well as providing opportunities for health education. Schools provide an opportunity to reach the pupils and their parents. The child to child programme is an example of how primary school children may take part in community based health education programmes such as the control of malaria and chlorination of wells.[5 6]

Who should do health education?

All health workers have a role in health education, and even if doctors and medical assistants have a large burden of clinical work they should regard patient education as an essential role (fig 2).[7] Since they are likely to be in overall charge of health centres and hospitals, they should take a lead in health education and in encouraging their staff—nursing, paramedical, and ancillary workers—to promote local health care and preventive policies. In most Third World countries there are too few trained health care workers but help may be enlisted from those who are already giving advice to the community—for example, public health workers, agricultural and community development officers, youth workers, home economists, adult literacy workers, and teachers. Such workers must, of course, be kept fully informed of health education programmes and given basic training on key health issues.

Village elders, religious leaders, traditional healers, and birth attendants often have considerable influence on their local community. The advice that they give may not, however, be correct and may contradict the policies advocated by the health workers. Then the health worker must seek out the leaders in the community and try to obtain their support. If this is gained they may be given a basic training under the supervision of the health centre and become the first tier of a primary health care service.[8]

How should health education be carried out?

Some of the characteristics of effective health education approaches are summarised in the box. A most useful method is to provide demonstrations where the advantages of adopting the recommended practices are clearly shown and the techniques and skills concerned may be practised. Such demonstrations will be helped if "satisfied users"—for example, successful users of oral rehydration, family planning, and breast feeding, as well as patients who have recovered from diseases such as leprosy—take part. All items used in demonstrations must be cheap and available locally; otherwise people will dismiss them as irrelevant to their situation.

Characteristics of effective health education

● Directed at people who have influence in the community

● Repeated and reinforced over time using different methods

● Adaptable, and uses existing channels of communication —for example, songs, drama, and story telling

● Entertaining and attracts the community's attention

● Uses clear simple language with local expressions and emphasises short term benefits of action

● Provides opportunities for dialogue and discussion to allow learner participation and feedback on understanding and implementation

● Uses demonstrations to show the benefits of adopting practices.

Word of mouth is perhaps the most valuable way to influence actions. Oral traditions in many rural societies are strong and people enjoy communication conveyed by means such as puppets, drama, story telling, and music. Wilson reports the use of parables and story telling to promote health education policies in Nigeria.[9] Songs and painted wall murals have been used in nutrition education in Uganda.[10] The traditional Caribbean calypso song has been used to promote family planning and oral rehydration solutions. Drama is emerging as one of the best ways of communicating both with urban and rural communities.[11] Using these folk media and drama may entail teaching the health worker new skills, and various manuals and teaching slide sets are available.[12-14] Local actors and musicians may themselves be prepared to use their skills to put over the message.

Finally, one to one education, small group discussion, and community meetings may provide opportunities for questions and discussion. Their effectiveness may be increased by using learning aids such as leaflets, charts, posters, flash cards, flip

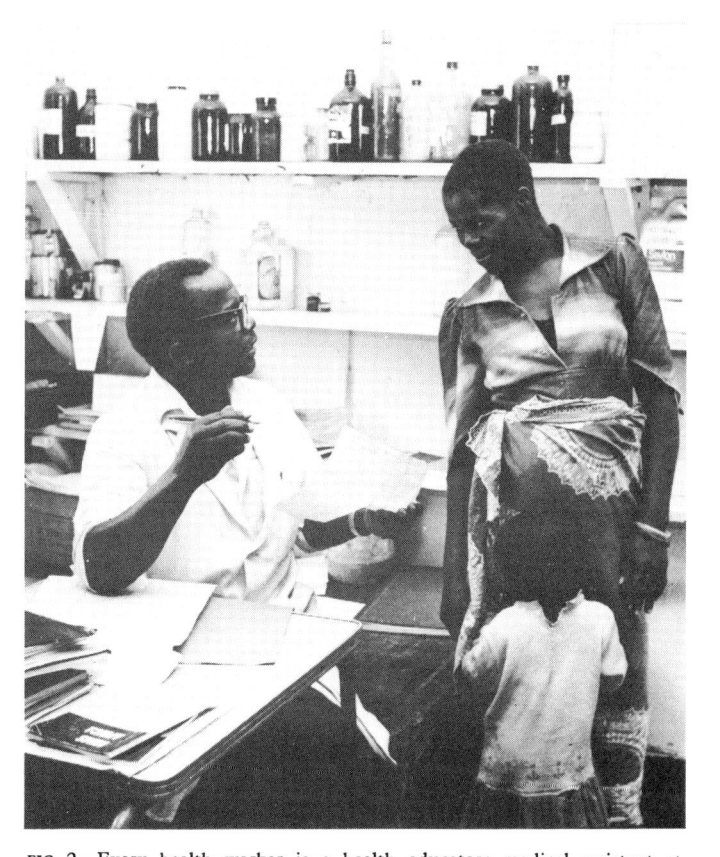

FIG 2—Every health worker is a health educator: medical assistant at Zambian rural health centre advising mother with child.

Principles of health education

charts, and flannelgraphs. Pictures need to be simple because many people will be unfamiliar with stylised Western pictures or biological diagrams.[15] It is a good idea to try out any leaflet or poster on members of the community to make sure they understand before circulating it more widely (fig 3). Films, slides, and film strips may be useful but have the disadvantage that projectors are expensive, and people may be so captivated by their novelty that they pay no attention to the content.

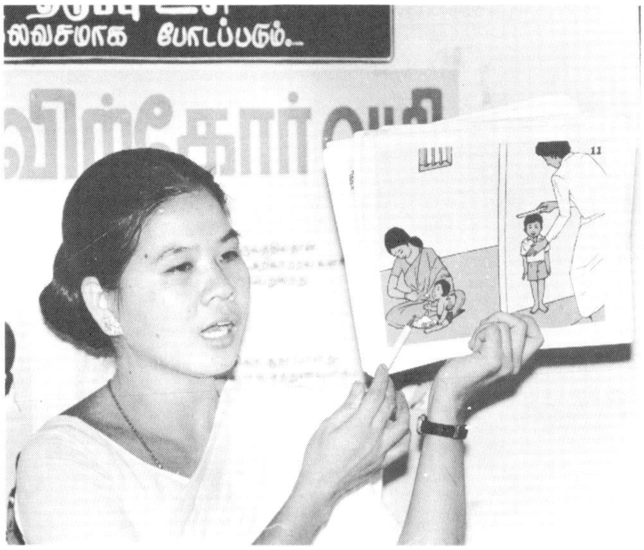

FIG 3—Audiovisual aids must be tried out to ensure that they are understood: health worker using flash cards in Tamil Nadu, South India.

The best way to use audiovisual aids is to draw people's attention and hold their interest while the health educator explains the important points. Leaflets are also useful, if the community is literate, to help people to remember the main points. The audience needs actively to take part in any discussion or demonstration and the educator can encourage this by asking questions and inviting comment. Flannelgraphs and a recent innovation of magnetised pictures on magnet boards are particularly good for encouraging participation.[17] Radio programmes are another good way to put over simple information related to large populations. Health information specific to the local community may be recorded on cassettes and played to small groups.[16] Details of many processes for producing simple low cost materials are reviewed in two excellent handbooks by Werner and Saunders.[12][18]

It is important to evaluate carefully the effectiveness of any health education activity, especially when new methods are being tried out. Evaluation can look for change in health status or practices. Other factors, however, can also be assessed, such as changes in beliefs, comprehension, population coverage, acceptability, and degree of community participation.

In planning any health education activity many failures can be prevented if communities are involved at the outset in the process of finding appropriate solutions to their health problems. This process of participation requires patient dialogue between health workers and communities. Although time consuming, this can yield many benefits in the long term through more relevant programmes and greater community involvement. Community participation is a key element of the emerging concept of primary health care as set out in the Alma Ata declaration of the World Health Organisation.

Leeds Polytechnic offers a specialist one year diploma course in health education in developing countries. Details of the course may be obtained from Dr J Hubley, Leeds Polytechnic, Calverley Street, Leeds LS1 3HE (tel 0532 462786).

References

1 Hubley JH. Making the community profile. *J Inst Health Educ* 1982;**20**:5-9.
2 Rogers EM. *Diffusion of innovations.* New York: The Free Press, 1983.
3 Church M. Value of traditional food practices. *J Hum Nut* 1976;**30**:9-12.
4 Laoye JA. Selling health in the market place. *World Health Forum* 1981;**2**:367-72.
5 Aarons A, Hawes H. *Child-to-child.* London and Basingstoke: Macmillan Press Ltd, 1979.
6 Joseph MV, Hubley JH. *Schools and primary health care.* Teaching slide set. St Albans: TALC (in press).
7 Brieger WR, Edozien, E. Pioneering patient education in Nigeria. *Africa Health* 1982/3; December/January:27-29.
8 Moynihan M, Kochar V, Sarma UC, *et al.* Training folk practitioners as PHWs in rural India. *Int J Health Educ* 1980;xxiii:167-78.
9 Hilton D. *Health teaching for West Africa.* Monograph Number 1, Wheaton, Illinois: MAP International, 1980. Available from TALC.
10 Church M. Health education and maternal and child health: newer considerations and international perspectives. In: Jelliffe DB, Jelliffe EFP, eds. *Advances in maternal and child health.* Vol 3. Oxford, Toronto, and New York: Oxford University Press, 1983:90-108.
11 Byram ML. Popular theatre as appropriate media. *Appropriate technology* 1980;**7**:21-2.
12 Werner D, Bower B. *Helping health workers learn.* Palo Alto California: Hesperian Foundation, 1982. Available from TALC.
13 Hesperian Foundation. *The measles monster.* Teaching slide set on drama and health education. Palo Alto: Hesperian Foundation.
14 Hesperian Foundation. *Puppets and dental health.* Teaching slide set. Palo Alto: Hesperian Foundation.
15 Moynihan M, Mukherjee U. Visual communication with non-literates: a review of current knowledge including research in northern India. *Int J Health Educ* 1981;xxiv:251-61.
16 Jenkins J. *Mass media for health education.* Cambridge: International Extension College, 1983.
17 *The Cassell visual learning system.* Visual Learning Division, Collier Macmillan, Suite 18, 91 St Martin's Lane, London WC2.
18 Saunders DJ. *Visual communication handbook: teaching and learning using simple visual materials.* Guildford: Lutterworths, 1979. Available from TALC.

Sources of information and audiovisual aids

Non-formal Education Information Centre, Michigan State University, East Lansing, Michigan 48824, USA.
TALC, Teaching Aids at Low Cost, Box 49, St Albans AL1 4AX, UK.
The Hesperian Foundation, PO Box 1692, Palo Alto, California 94302, USA.

Recommended reading

HYGIE (formerly *Int J Health Education*), 9 Rue Newton F-75116 Paris, France.
Education for Health. WHO, Avenue Appia, 1211 Geneva 27, Switzerland.
International Quarterly of Community Health Education. Baywood Publ Co, 120 Marine Street, PO Box D, Farmingdale NY 11735, USA.

APPROPRIATE TEACHING AIDS

DAVID MORLEY,   FELICITY SAVAGE KING

When health workers from a developing country visit a national or international "centre of excellence," they may feel frustrated rather than helped. They realise that they have no access to high technology books, journals, films, and slides, or to the new ideas on how to use them. This discovery may prompt doubts about their ability to do their work in the absence of such props. Some are tempted to abandon their posts altogether and look for a solution in academic activity. This happens so often that there is a steady drain of skilled people from the health service periphery to the centre—regionally, nationally, and internationally. This flow needs to be reversed, and those who work at the centres should share their knowledge and resources with those who work in the periphery. Relevant, practical, up to date, and inexpensive books and other teaching materials need to reach district training schools and community health workers. In addition, it is essential to ensure that people know how to use them.

Appropriate teaching materials

The teaching materials that are needed include books, newsletters, films, flannelgraphs, and colour slides. Of these, books are the most important because they are durable and require no equipment to use. Western medical books adopt a theoretical or systematic approach, and use technical and grammatically complex academic language. Any practical instructions that they include are frequently incomplete and may be difficult to extract. Primary health care workers with limited secondary education, who use English only as a second language, may find such books impossible to read. Thus there is a need for appropriate health training books, which was first recognised in the late 1960s.[1] Nevertheless, it was not until the early 1970s that Cripwell and colleagues worked out in detail what syntax second language English speakers could and could not understand easily.[2] Recent publications have extended their techniques and the information is presented in simple language with short, active sentences, and limited vocabulary.[3] A page of solid print may be daunting so it is advisable to break it up with lists, slogans, titled paragraphs, and illustrations, which may improve understanding and are often remembered long after the text is forgotten. Both these features are shown in two recent books by David Werner.[4,5]

Cost is a major consideration, but if a book is subsidised at publication the cost to the reader may be kept down to about £2 (0·5p to 1p per page), and experience has shown that peripheral health workers buy books that are made available to them at this price.[6-8] Import and currency restrictions may limit the availability of books—local reprinting may help to overcome this. Organisations that distribute books at low cost include TALC (Teaching Aids at Low Cost), and the Voluntary Health Association of India.

NEWSLETTERS

Short, simply produced newsletters may provide up to date information and continuing education. They have the advantages of providing information in small doses, and they are easy to read and very helpful for isolated health workers who may not be able to obtain or afford up to date books. Several newsletters are sent free anywhere in the world to anyone who sends in their address and a request—for example, *Diarrhoea Dialogue*.[9] Locally produced journals, such as *Afya* in Kenya, and *Bwino* in Zambia, help to fill local needs, and even more locally based duplicated newsletters, such as *Shasta Barta*, for a community health programme in Bangladesh, help to keep isolated health workers in touch with others in their own programme.[10]

LOCALLY PRODUCED BOOKS

Locally produced books are needed to overcome cultural barriers as well as trade restrictions. Books that are written in another country may not be appropriate for local needs. Isolated health care workers need straightforward texts that are written in the local language, with simple illustrations that include people with local facial features, clothing, and implements. Books produced internationally are more likely to be useful as reference works for translation and adaptation. An example of what may be achieved is provided by a community health programme in Guinea

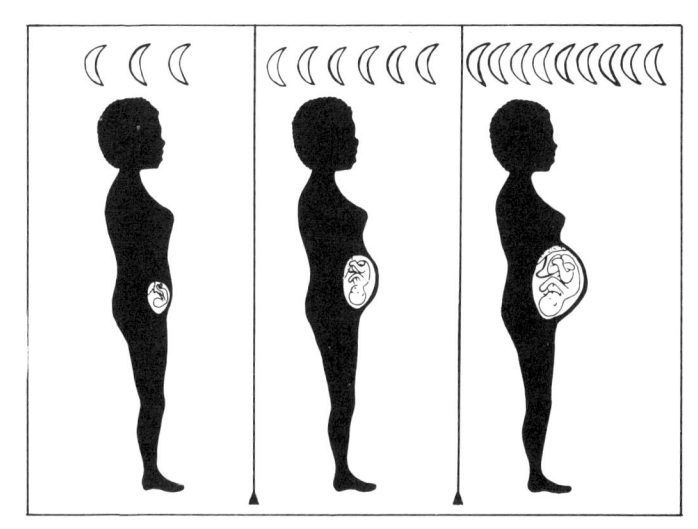

FIG 1—Picture symbol used to teach community health workers about pregnancy in Guinea Bissau.[11]

Appropriate teaching aids

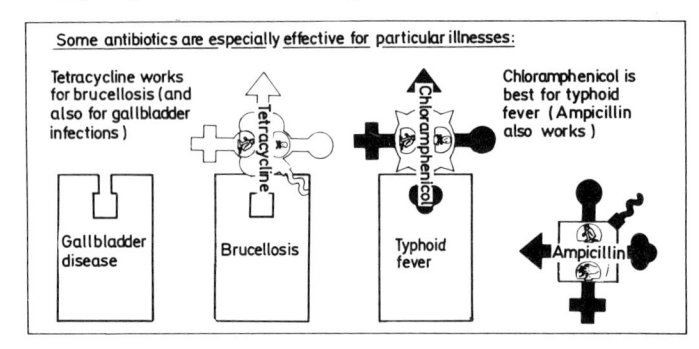

FIG 2—Picture symbols to teach health workers about antibiotics, from *Helping Health Workers Learn*.[5]

Bissau that trains completely illiterate village health workers. They have achieved this by producing very simple pictorial training materials and by using picture symbols instead of words, both for training and to label containers of medicine.[11] Many other valuable training ideas are included in *Helping Health Workers Learn*.[5] To take an example, simple symbols cut out of cardboard may be used to teach village health workers the use of antibiotics. The authors found that after two days' playing with these symbols village health workers understood the use of antibiotics better than some doctors.

SLIDES

Colour slides are extremely popular with health workers, because they may short circuit the struggle to describe things in words, and show exactly what the teacher means. They are, however, suited only to students who have had some secondary education. Slides have several advantages over films. They are cheaper and require simpler projectors, and they are more flexible because the teacher may select and arrange the material to suit his or her own lecture and to go at his or her own speed. Slides may be used with a prepared tape, but they are probably best used with a printed text. The teacher should use the text as a guide and source of ideas, rather than as a set lecture. TALC has been particularly successful in developing and distributing sets of slides, on over 60 topics. The material is supplied at minimal cost: 24 slides together with a detailed text and teaching guide and a small plastic viewer, and including postage and packing, all cost less than half the price of a new colour film.

FILMS

Although films are popular as entertainment, many teachers have become disillusioned with them as teaching aids. They are expensive, and each copy may be used only about 30 times. They aim at a wide audience, so that they may not be locally relevant, and the teacher cannot control the speed of delivery. It is difficult and expensive to maintain a film projector in a hot, dusty climate, and in some rural areas annual maintenance may cost as much as the original equipment. Video productions may eventually replace films because the cost of production and of duplication is much less.

FLANNELGRAPHS

Flannelgraphs have proved useful for teaching health workers about growth charts and for putting over simple messages in the villages. TALC distributes a growth chart kit, which includes a yellow flannel background chart, and a moveable calendar of months, dots, and labels to put on to the background. To teach health workers to fill them in, you need cheap duplicated paper growth charts for each student. A precut stencil to help you to

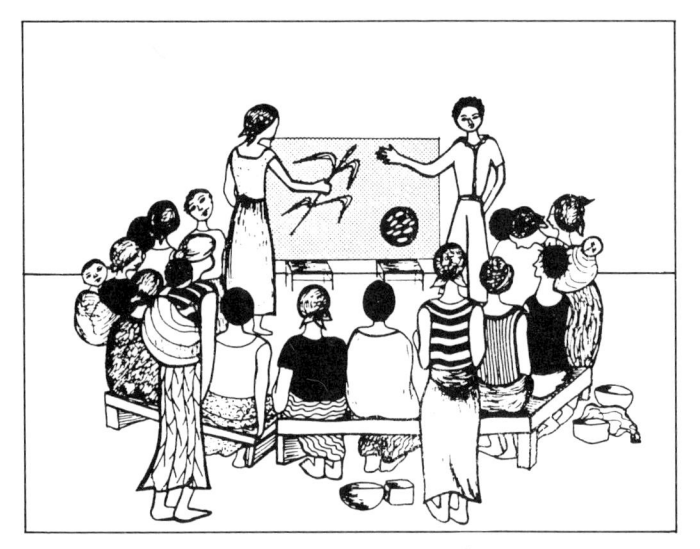

FIG 3—Flannelgraph for health education of the public.[12]

prepare these is included in the kit. To aid interpretation, you need either slides or a flannelgraph, or both. You cannot satisfactorily draw a growth chart on the blackboard. Flannelgraphs are also useful for health education of the public. You can build up a story on a flannel board, using pictures which have either cloth or sandpaper on the back. The pictures must show local objects as far as possible. For this reason, these materials often need to be locally produced. A flannelgraph for teaching child health and nutrition has been widely used in west Africa, and to this has now been added a flannelgraph on helminths. Both of these are designed for use at village level.[12] Another important health education medium is drama, whether acted by people, as in Nigeria,[13] or by puppets, such as the "wayang kulit" of Indonesia.

The future

During the past 20 years there have been great developments in our ideas about health, and these are matched by similar developments in ideas about education. Bringing health workers in from remote stations to somewhere more central for refresher training is expensive and has the effect of reducing what may already be a limited peripheral health service. Thus few courses are arranged, and, when they are, they include senior rather than junior workers. A distance learning programme (working on the principle of the Open University in the United Kingdom) could train the whole health team and provide a continuing training programme for health workers who have had practical experience of the problems that they are expected to deal with and need some feedback. Above all, distance learning is a way to get ideas about how to improve health outside academic institutions and in the community.

References

1 King MH, King FMA, Morley DC, Burgess HLJ, Burgess AP. *Nutrition for developing countries*. Oxford: Oxford University Press, 1972.
2 Savage F, Godwin P. Controlling your language: making English clear. *Trans R Soc Trop Med Hyg* 1981;75:583–5.
3 King MH, King FMA, Martodipoero S. *Primary child care*. Oxford: Oxford University Press, 1978.
4 Werner D. *Where there is no doctor*. Palo Alto, California: The Hesperian Foundation, 1977.
5 Werner D, Bower B. *Helping health workers learn*. Palo Alto, California: The Hesperian Foundation, 1982.
6 Morley D, Rohde J, Williams G. *Practising health for all*. Oxford: Oxford University Press, 1983.
7 Cameron M, Hofvander Y. *Manual on feeding infants and young children*. Oxford: Oxford University Press, 1983.
8 Helsing E, Savage King F. *Breast feeding in practice*. Oxford: Oxford University Press, 1982.

Appropriate teaching aids

9 Appropriate Health Resources and Technologies Action Group. *Diarrhoea Dialogue*. London: AHRTAG. (A list of other free newsletters about health will be sent on request to TALC, address see below).
10 Schweiger M. *A community worker's newsletter*. TALC slide set, 1984.
11 Chabot J. *A community health project in Africa*. TALC slide set, 1984.
12 Gordon G, Gordon S. *Nutrition and child health flannelgraph*. Available from TALC, 1982.
13 Hilton D. "Tell us a story": health teaching in Nigeria. In: Morley D, Rohde J, Williams G, eds. *Practising health for all*. Oxford: Oxford University Press, 1983.

Organisations mentioned in the text

TALC, Teaching Aids at Low Cost, Administrator: Mrs B Harvey, Box 49, St Albans AL1 4AX, UK.

VHAI, Voluntary Health Association of India, C-14 Community Centre, Safdarjung Development Area, New Delhi 110016, India.

AMREF, African Medical and Research Foundation, Box 30125, Nairobi, Kenya.

The Hesperian Foundation, Box 1692, Palo Alto, CA 94302, USA.

AHRTAG Appropriate Health Resources Technology Action Group, 85 Marylebone High Street, London W1M 3DE, UK.

MENTAL HEALTH CARE IN THE DISTRICT HOSPITAL

H G EGDELL

Psychiatric disorders are not peculiar to Western countries, and within the community served by a district general hospital in the Third World the incidence of major mental illness is about 1%; furthermore, the risk of any individual developing such a disorder is 10%.[1] Other studies in the developing world have found that 5-20% of patients have some form of psychiatric illness—commonly anxiety and depression—which may present with a variety of physical symptoms.[2] Few district hospitals have specialist psychiatric facilities or trained staff. This means that general duties doctors may have to take responsibility for providing care for patients with psychiatric illness. Help from the nursing and other health care workers is essential, although their co-operation may be difficult to obtain because of ignorance about, and prejudice towards, mental illness. My decision to initiate psychiatric visits to an upcountry hospital in Uganda was at first met with suspicion by the doctors, who thought that they would have to admit disruptive patients to their wards. Nevertheless, I received a warm welcome from medical assistants who were seeking help in the management of outpatients with somatic symptoms of anxiety and depression.

If psychiatric care is to be undertaken by general medical staff they must be familiar with modern psychiatric treatment and take the lead in preparing the other members of the hospital staff, and support them through their initial anxieties in looking after patients with psychiatric illness. It is also essential that priorities for care should be defined. Thus if Morley's guidelines are adopted those conditions that are common, disabling, disturbing, and treatable must be identified.[3] In a study in seven developing countries community representatives, health staff, and research teams selected psychiatric emergencies (acute psychosis, suicide attempts, drug and alcohol abuse), grand mal epilepsy, and chronic psychosis as their priorities.[4]

Management of psychiatric emergencies

Community leaders and village health workers have no problems in identifying patients with psychoses.[5] Many languages have their own words for the "run mad" and the "quietly mad"—for example, eddalu and l'akalogojjo in Uganda.[6 7] Probably, however, treatment will be sought only when the patient is acutely disturbed or if a hospital shows a particular interest or success in treating such patients. Acute psychoses often present with unacceptable behaviour such as abuse, going naked, overactivity, and destructiveness. The patient may arrive at the hospital tied up, handcuffed, or fastened to a large log of wood. Whatever the circumstances it is important to obtain a good history from the relatives, the local headman, or the police. In particular seek evidence of physical illness, including epilepsy, ask about alcohol and drug intake, and establish whether the patient is always fully aware of his surroundings and orientated in time, place, and person.

Patients often cooperate with the doctor given the opportunity. I once met a naked young man handcuffed to a hospital bed, which he dragged behind him through the hospital compound, waving a large stone in his free hand. The nursing staff had formed a wary circle around him. On being asked his problem the patient complained of too many injections in his buttock. After a further talk and a mug of tea he accepted a large injection of largactil into his arm. This anecdote illustrates that the staff's natural anxiety may actually encourage the patient's disturbed behaviour.

If faced with a violent patient keep calm and ensure that two or three male staff or relatives are near but not too close to be intimidating. Tell the patient that the staff are there to protect him from harm (from himself or others) and encourage him to talk. Offer food and drink but leave him plenty of "personal space." If he remains disturbed and overactive offer chlorpromazine 50-100 mg orally to help him "feel better and be in control." If he is cooperative arrange admission to a quiet room with minimal furnishings. Some hospital staff have an intuitive skill in calming the disturbed, and it is important to appreciate that time spent waiting for the patient to decide to accept treatment is more productive than a hasty attempt to overwhelm him. Physical restraint is rarely necessary and should be used only if violence persists. The aim of such restraint is to prevent the patient harming either himself or others and to administer a tranquilliser. It is best achieved by holding the patient's clothes, shoulders, mid-thighs, and calves, keeping the legs together and avoiding putting pressure on the neck, chest, or abdomen. The patient is then forced to lie face down on the mattress or floor. Remove any objects that may cause injury, such as shoes. Talk to the patient continuously, telling him when, where, and why the injection is being given. Chlorpromazine 100 mg intramuscularly (less if the patient is small or elderly) is effective and may be repeated every two hours. When oral medication is accepted the dose may be doubled, and the maintenance dose should be 200 mg (or less) four times a day. Haloperidol 5-10 mg intramuscularly half to one hourly (depending on size and age) followed by 10-20 mg given orally four times a day is an alternative regimen.[8] These drugs may cause excessive sedation and hypotension, but the commonest error is to give an inadequate dose for too short a time.

Drug treatment has largely replaced electroconvulsive therapy. Two 60 bed provincial psychiatric units in Kenya have not used electroconvulsive therapy for over 18 months (Acuda, personal communication). On rare occasions, however, patients with resistant severe psychotic depression or uncontrollable excitement may need electroconvulsive therapy, and for this they should be referred to a specialised psychiatric unit.

Making a diagnosis

ORGANIC ILLNESS

Any patient who presents in an acutely disturbed state must be

Mental health care in the district hospital

examined and investigated to exclude organic disease. The history is also very important, and evidence of clouding of consciousness, disorientation, impaired thinking and memory, and marked anxiety with a fluctuating general state must be sought. Minor impairment of memory may be established only by questioning about recent events and asking the patient to remember a name and address after five minutes. Visual hallucinations are common in organic psychosis. Table I serves as a guide to the aetiology of acute organic reactions. The doctor should be particularly aware of the common local diseases, and in this respect it is of interest to note that the two most commonly used drugs in Butabika Mental Hospital, Uganda, were chlorpromazine and chloramphenicol. This was due to the misdiagnosis of typhoid as a functional psychosis.

TABLE I—*Causes of acute organic reactions. (Reproduced from W A Lishman's* Organic Psychiatry[39] *by kind permission)*

	Symptoms
(1) Degenerative	Presenile or senile dementias complicated by infection, anoxia, etc
(2) Space occupying lesions	Cerebral tumour, subdural haematoma, cerebral abscess
(3) Trauma	"Acute post-traumatic psychosis"
(4) Infection	Encephalitis, meningitis, subacute meningovascular syphilis. Exanthemas, streptococcal infection, septicaemia, pneumonia, influenza, typhoid, typhus, cerebral malaria, trypanosomiasis, rheumatic chorea
(5) Vascular	Acute cerebral thrombosis or embolism, episode in arteriosclerotic dementia, transient cerebral ischaemic attack, subarachnoid haemorrhage, hypertensive encephalopathy, systemic lupus erythematosus
(6) Epileptic	Psychomotor seizures, petit mal status, postictal states
(7) Metabolic	Uraemia, liver disorder, electrolyte disturbances, alkalosis, acidosis, hypercapnia, remote effects of carcinoma, porphyria
(8) Endocrine	Hyperthyroid crises, myxoedema, Addisonian crises, hypopituitarism, hypoparathyroidism and hyperparathyroidism, diabetic pre-coma, hypoglycaemia
(9) Toxic	Alcohol: Wernicke's encephalopathy, delirium tremens. Drugs: barbiturates (including withdrawal), bromides, salicylate intoxication, cannabis, LSD, prescribed medications (antiparkinsonian drugs, scopalamine, tricyclic and monoamine oxidase inhibitor antidepressants, digoxin, etc). Others: lead, arsenic, organic mercury compounds, carbon disulphide
(10) Anoxia	Bronchopneumonia, congestive cardiac failure, cardiac arrhythmias, silent coronary infarction, silent bleeding, carbon monoxide poisoning, post-anaesthetic
(11) Vitamin deficiency	Thiamine (Wernicke's encephalopathy), nicotinic acid (pellagra, acute nicotinic-acid-deficient encephalopathy, B_{12} and folic acid deficiency

FUNCTIONAL (NON-ORGANIC) PSYCHOSIS

Schizophrenia with delusions of special powers or persecution out of keeping with local beliefs, and auditory hallucinations, may present with or without excitement. The manic patient is overactive, sleepless, and disinhibited with euphoria and grandiose ideas. Such patients need to be carefully examined for evidence of physical illness once their excitement has been controlled. Chlorpromazine 50-200 mg four times a day or haloperidol 10-20 mg four times a day, reducing slowly to smaller maintenance doses depending on response, usually provides satisfactory control. Stress induced psychosis is common in developing countries. It may follow adverse life events such as bereavement or assault, but more subtle personal precipitants may be difficult to identify. Most patients with acute psychoses settle rapidly and medication may be withdrawn slowly. Those with persisting symptoms—usually chronic schizophrenia (which has a better outlook than in Western countries)—may need maintenance doses of major tranquillisers. Depot preparations such as fluphenazine decanoate 25-100 mg intramuscularly or flupenthixol 40-120 mg intramuscularly every three or four weeks may overcome problems of compliance with oral treatment. These preparations are expensive but are cheaper than repeated admissions to hospital.[9] It is advisable to keep a register of patients receiving maintenance treatment so that a failure to attend for further treatment and review may alert staff to take action to prevent a disruptive relapse.

Acute alcoholic psychoses (delirium tremens) may be controlled by a benzodiazepine—for example, diazepam 50-75 mg daily reducing after two or three days and stopping in a week. Haloperidol is an alternative. These patients and their families will need counselling on the hazards of excess drink and the benefits of reduced intake. Patients with epilepsy may also present with acute psychosis, which usually implies poor compliance with anticonvulsant treatment. Follow up should include supervision of medication as well as counselling of the patients and their relatives.

Management of patients with neuroses

A survey of 1624 outpatients in primary care clinics in four developing countries showed an overall frequency of psychiatric illness of 13·9%—mainly the physical symptoms of anxiety and depression.[10 11] More than 20% of outpatients who complained of weakness, dizziness, or abdominal or chest pain had a psychiatric disorder. Those with three or more symptoms were twice as likely to be mentally ill. These patients make huge demands on the hospital staff and on the hospital budget because many undergo needless investigations. In my view, the general duties doctor must be prepared to assess and when necessary treat these patients, and to do this he must be attuned to looking for depression, stress reactions, the anxiety aspects of physical illness, and the chronic symptoms of the anxiety prone individual.[12]

Patients with depressive illness may not complain of depression, but there are cross cultural core symptoms of sadness, joylessness, anxiety, tension, lack of energy, loss of interests, loss of concentration, and ideas of insufficiency, inadequacy, and worthlessness.[13] Antidepressants such as amitriptyline 25-75 mg twice daily may be very effective in these patients. In patients with anxiety, however, the doctor's first task is to help them understand that their condition has psychosocial rather than disease origins. Appropriate adjustments to their way of life may then become apparent. The doctor must promote self help and guide the patients towards tackling their own problems. Techniques of relaxation, desensitisation, implosion therapy, and brief psychotherapy with clear, feasible objectives may help the doctor to deal with patients who are often demanding and difficult to treat.[14 15] Minor tranquillisers such as diazepam and chlordiazepoxide should be used to treat only acute, severely disabling, short lived anxiety. They cannot solve psychosocial problems, and Third World health services cannot afford to follow the widespread and largely ineffective use of minor tranquillisers that has been evident in Western countries.

Patients who deliberately harm themselves or attempt suicide must be asssessed carefully. Underlying psychosis or severe depression needs to be treated and all cases need close supervision while the underlying stresses on the patients and their family are assessed. It may be helpful to refer patients to community or religious leaders or, in some cases, traditional healers, who can provide further support and counselling. Nursing staff and primary health workers seldom have the time or the necessary skills to provide specialised care for such patients.

Attitudes to mental health

Mental health is now part of modern training programmes, but many hospital staff are still not yet prepared to manage patients with psychiatric disorders, especially those with neuroses, which were given a low priority in recent recommendations by the World Health Organisation.[16] I think that this is regrettable, especially with respect to depressive illness, which is common, easy to recognise, and treatable. In my view a major change in attitudes and allocation of resources to meet the needs of the mentally ill is needed. The first step could be to set up a local workshop where health staff could meet community and religious leaders, members of voluntary associations, teachers, and other interested persons to clarify priority problems and consider a community response to these. On an assignment in Swaziland, funded by the World Health Organisation, I found that the rural health motivators (mature and respected individuals with three months' general health training) grasped psychosocial concepts rapidly and were keen to help patients. Simple counselling skills could prepare them for potentially valuable work with outpatients, especially healthy young people who present with non-specific complaints such as eye strain, poor concentration, and academic failure. A manual for the

Mental health care in the district hospital

disabled has been published recently and has many other suggestions for community action.[17]

Some traditional healers specialise in mental health,[18 19] but does this mean that the doctor should cooperate with them? I believe that the wide variations in skill among such individuals must lead the doctor to be cautious, and that he should make a careful local assessment of their skills, methods of treatment, and results before committing himself to any formal liaison. It is salutary to remember, however, that patients will attend these healers anyway, both before and after they receive their Western care, regardless of the doctor's views.

Problems in childhood

Primary health care workers in the Sudan, Philippines, India, and Colombia have reported mental health problems in 12-29% of children seen.[20] Symptoms that are inconsistent, unusual, or associated with special circumstances are helpful pointers to diagnosis, as is the opinion of the attending adult.[21] Hyperkinesis may be associated with brain damage, developmental problems, or family problems.[22 23] Amphetamine up to 30 mg daily may help, though small doses of chlorpromazine, slowly increasing to 50 to 100 mg daily, may be all that is available. The attitudes of the family and school are crucial. Hysteria, manifested for example as aphonia or paralysis without physical illness, usually follows stress, though details may need tactful exploration. Admission to hospital may allow a face saving recovery while the underlying stress factors are explored and ameliorated. Nocturnal enuresis has been managed effectively by parents in Swaziland by ignoring wetting and rewarding dry nights using star charts (Guinness, personal communication). Similar management of encopresis is possible.[24] Care of children with epilepsy must include measures to overcome negative attitudes in the community.

Mental handicap is considered to be untreatable by some doctors, but communities have placed it high on their priorities for care.[4] Parents lose heart and fail to teach domestic and self care skills, and unsatisfactory habits are established. A simple approach is to start with the control of fits or hyperkinesis and then teach that the mentally handicapped can learn but that they do so slowly. Various techniques have been devised for family use.[17] A scheme using mothers and village aides as teachers of mentally handicapped children is proving successful in Kenya (Horsfield, personal communication).

Training

The doctor in a Third World district hospital should initiate training schemes for health staff concentrating on a few tasks that are seen as priorities—for example, the use of drugs, restraint of the violent patient, and community care. Ask the country's psychiatrists and health teachers to visit the hospital for joint discussions with local health trainers and to take part in teaching the staff and arranging workshops. Brief psychiatric secondment for selected health staff is feasible in some countries—for example, in Bangladesh regular courses are run for district hospital doctors (Dr Hidayetal Islam, professor of psychiatry, Dacca). Zambia has a well established training scheme for medical assistants, which was started by Professor Alan Haworth. In India a similar approach has potentially wider application.[25] Further ideas may be gleaned by reviewing local pilot systems of care.[26 27] Training manuals may be most helpful, and several have been produced.[28-34] The use of flow charts is another valuable way to teach health workers.[35]

It is useful to compile a list of psychotropic drugs that are available in the hospital, together with standard dose regimens (table II). A local glossary of psychiatric terms is also helpful together with a list of local interpreters who need a brief training in how to elicit a psychiatric history. The use of non-hospital staff implies that policy decisions should be made to sanction their participation in the care of patients with psychiatric disorders. Their responsibilities and training will require the cooperation of local and probably national health trainers. Finally, the success of any training programmes should be evaluated.[36-38]

TABLE II—*Recommended psychotropic drugs for district general hospitals (second choices in parentheses)*

Chlorpromazine {25 mg, 100 mg tablet / 25 mg/ml injection}
Haloperidol 5 mg tablet
Fluphenazine decanoate 25 mg/ml injection
(Trifluoperazine 5 mg tablet)
(Flupenthixol decanoate 20 mg/ml injection)
Procyclidine 5 mg tablet
Diazepam 5 mg tablet
Amitriptyline 25 mg tablet
(Imipramine 25 mg tablet)
(Lithium carbonate 250 mg tablet)
(Mianserin and Nomifensine are antidepressants with fewer side effects but very expensive)

Health staff will need guidance sheets.

Conclusion

The general duties doctor can provide effective mental health care in a district hospital. Although psychoses usually take precedence over neuroses, local priorities of care must be identified. Intervention and appropriate management of these disorders may be achieved with limited facilities and scant resources.[16] The most important hurdle may well be that of overcoming local ignorance and prejudice.

I thank Mrs Irene Tierney for secretarial help and Mrs Betty O'Brien and Mrs Dorothy Howard for help with references.

References

1 World Health Organisation. Organisation of mental health services in developing countries. *WHO Tech Rep Ser* 1975;No 564.
2 Egdell HG. Mental health care in the developing world. Brief review of first phase of WHO collaborative study on strategies for extending mental health care. *Trop Doct* 1983;13:149-52.
3 Morley D. *Paediatric priorities in the developing world*. London: Butterworth, 1973.
4 Climent CE, Diop BSM, Harding TW, Ibrahim HHA, Ladrido-Ignacio L, Wig NN. Mental health in primary health care. *WHO Chron* 1980;34:231-6.
5 Wig NN, Suleiman MA, Routledge R, et al. Community reactions to mental disorders: a key informant study in three developing countries. *Acta Psychiatr Scand* 1980;61:111-26.
6 Orley JH. *Culture and mental illness: a study from Uganda*. Nairobi: East African Publishing House, 1970.
7 Edgerton RB. Conceptions of psychosis in four east African societies. *American Anthropologist* 1966;68:408-25.
8 Donlon PT, Hopkin J, Tupin JP. Overview: efficacy and safety of rapid neuroleptization method with injectable haloperidol. *Am J Psychiatry* 1979;136:273-8.
9 Brook MG. Community care programme for chronic psychotic patients on a small Caribbean island. *Trop Doct* (in press).
10 Harding TW, de Arango MV, Baltazar J, et al. Mental disorders in primary health care: a study of their frequency and diagnosis in four developing countries. *Psychol Med* 1980;10:231-41.
11 Harding TW, Climent CE, Diop M, et al. The WHO collaborative study on strategies for extending mental health care. II. The development of new research methods. *Am J Psychiatry* 1983;140:1474-80.
12 Acuda W, Egdell HG. Anxiety and depression and the general doctor. *Trop Doct* 1984;14:51-5.
13 Sartorius N, Jablensky A, Gulbinat W, Ernberg G. WHO collaborative study: assessment of depressive disorders. *Psychol Med* 1980;10:743-9.
14 Wilkinson JCM, Latif K. *Behaviour therapy*. Derby, England: Pastures Hospital, 1972.
15 Bloch S, ed. *An introduction to the psychotherapies*. Oxford: Oxford Medical Publications, 1979.
16 Harding TW, Busnello Ed'A, Climent CE, et al. The WHO collaborative study on strategies for extending mental health care. III. Evaluative design and illustrative results. *Am J Psychiatry* 1983;140:1481-5.
17 Helander E, Mendis P, Nelson G. *Training disabled people in the community. A manual on community-based rehabilitation for developing countries*. Geneva: WHO, 1983. (RHB/83.1.)
18 Green EC. Roles for African traditional healers in mental health care. *Medical Anthropology* 1980; autumn:489-522.
19 Kapur R. The role of traditional healers in mental health care in rural India. *Indian Social Science and Medicine* 1979;13B:27-31.
20 Giel R, de Arango MV, Climent CE, et al. Childhood mental disorders in primary health care: results of observations in four developing countries. *Pediatrics* 1981;68:677-83.
21 Egdell HG. Problem children and the general doctor. *Trop Doct* 1984;14:103-7.
22 Egdell HG, Stanfield JP. Paediatric neurology in Africa: a Ugandan report. *Br Med J* 1972;i:548-52.
23 Kolvin I, Goodyer I. Child psychiatry. In: Granville-Grossman K, ed. *Recent advances in clinical psychiatry 4*. London: Churchill Livingstone, 1982:1-24.
24 Kolvin I, Macmillan A. Child psychiatry. In: Granville-Grossman K, ed. *Recent advances in clinical psychiatry 2*. London: Churchill Livingstone, 1976:296-350.
25 Murthy RS, Wig NN. The WHO collaborative study on strategies for extending mental health care. IV. A training approach to enhancing the availability of mental health manpower in a developing country. *Am J Psychiatry* 1983;140:1486-90.
26 Wig NN, Murthy RS, Harding TW. A model for rural psychiatric services—Raipur Rani experience. *Indian Journal of Psychiatry* 1981;23:275-90.
27 Baasher T, El-Hakim A, Galat A, Habbashy E. Rural psychiatry: the Fayoum experiment. *Egypt J Psychiatry* 1979;2:77-87.
28 Wankiiri VB. *Training manual for identification and management of mental health problems (for mid-level primary health workers)*. Geneva: WHO.
29 Wankiiri VB. *Mental health module (student text). Rural health development project*. Maseru, Lesotho: Ministry of Health and Social Welfare, 1982.
30 Wankiiri VB. *Community mental health care—a manual for health workers*. Geneva: WHO, 1982.
31 Swift CR. *Mental health: a manual for medical assistants and other rural health workers*. Nairobi: African Medical and Research Foundation, 1977.
32 Murphy RS. Mental health component of primary health care manuals—a review. *Journal of the National Institute of Mental Health and Neurosciences, Bangalore, India* 1983;1:91-8.

33 Ladrigo-Ignacio L, Climent CE, de Arango MV, Baltazar J. Research screening instruments as tools in training health workers for mental health care. *Trop Geogr Med* 1983;35:1-7.
34 World Health Organisation. *A manual on child mental health and psychosocial development. I. For the primary health care physician. II. For the primary health worker. III. For teachers. IV. For workers in children's homes.* New Delhi: WHO, 1982.
35 Essex B, Gosling H. *Programme for identification and management of mental health problems.* (Tropical health series.) Edinburgh and London: Churchill Livingstone, 1982.
36 World Health Organisation. Mental health care in developing countries: a critical appraisal of research findings. *WHO Tech Rep Ser* 1984;No 698.
37 Hassler FR. Evaluation of mental health services. In: Baasher TA, Carstairs GM, Giel R, Hassler FR, eds. *Mental health services in developing countries.* Geneva: WHO, 1975.
38 World Health Organisation. *Managerial process for national health development.* Geneva: WHO, 1981.
39 Lishman WA. *Organic psychiatry. The psychological consequences of cerebral disorder.* Oxford: Blackwell Scientific, 1978:182-3.

Suggestions for further reading

Tropical Doctor: Issues July 1983 to April 1985 contain a series of articles on the recognition and management of mental illness in adults and children for the general doctor working independently and far from advanced medical centres.

Asuni T, Swift CR. *Psychiatry in an African setting.* (Mental health: rural health series.) Nairobi: African Medical Research Foundation, 1977.

Swift CR. *Mental health: a manual for medical assistants and other rural health workers.* Nairobi: African Medical and Research Foundation, 1977.

Barker P. *Basic child psychiatry.* 4th ed. London: Granada, 1983. (Paperback £7·95.) Principles and practice that can be adapted to the Third World.

Essex B, Gosling H. *Programme for identification and management of mental health problems.* (Tropical health series.) Edinburgh and London: Churchill Livingstone, 1982. (Softback £2·30.) Carefully evaluated and practical flow charts especially useful in teaching health staff who will work in isolation.

World Health Organisation. Organisation of mental health services in developing countries. *WHO Tech Rep Ser* 1975;No 564. Basic document for all health teachers and administrators.

World Health Organisation. Mental health care in developing countries: a critical appraisal of research findings. *WHO Tech Rep Ser* 1984;No 698.

The following publications illustrate that mental health is a broad, positive concept and not simply the absence of mental illness. They are helpful in provoking staff to think beyond hospital walls.

World Health Organisation. *Promoting health in the human environment.* Geneva: WHO, 1975.
World Health Organisation. *Social dimensions of mental health.* Geneva: WHO, 1981.

WRITING IT DOWN

PAUL SNELL

In medical practice it is all too easy to drown in paperwork or, at the other extreme, to jeopardise the results of a job well done by leaving vital facts unrecorded. In developing countries it is particularly necessary to avoid wasting time and making inaccurate or unnecessary records, so what are the arguments in favour of keeping medical records? What is the best form on which to record information? Who should record the information? And, finally, who should keep the records?

Why keep records?

Records are needed to aid management of individual patients and for obtaining information for epidemiological purposes. The latter was the subject of Dr Peter Cox's article (p 29), so in this article I will concentrate on the requirements for individual patient management. In my view records serve three purposes, which may be reflected in separate documents or combined as described here:

(1) To give to whoever may attend the patient at an accident the bare essentials that may prove useful for emergency treatment.

(2) To give to the patient (or his family or friend) information that he needs to play his part in restoring or maintaining his health.

(3) To remind or inform the doctor (or other health worker) of the diagnosis, medical history, previous investigations, etc, so that at any future encounter information on what has previously been found and done is readily available.

Which form?

The conflict in keeping good medical records lies between completeness and accessibility. The most complete may be an encyclopaedic dossier that is filed in the bowels of a teaching hospital. The simplest is a scar or tattoo—accessible but very limited. Other considerations include the time and skill required to complete the record, its accuracy and confidentiality. The ideal solution to good record keeping will vary because of the widely different circumstances of district hospitals in the Third World. Nevertheless, the system described below may prove of interest. It was devised (after drawing on many people's ideas,[1] and with some juggling and refining over 15 years) in a mission hospital in the Ivory Coast. The work of the hospital and its health workers included providing an extended village programme, and many hundreds of patients were seen each day.

WALLET CARD FOR THE BARE ESSENTIALS

For a card to have any chance of being read at the scene of an accident it must be brief, and it should be kept with the identity card in those countries that have them. The essential items to include are: blood group; state of tetanus immunisation (and advice concerning boosters or serum in case the victim has dirty wounds); allergies; relevant medical disorders—for example, diabetes—and regular medication—for example, steroids. Nevertheless, the cards may not be read and, even if they are, may not be acted on, so their value needs to be assessed with a degree of scepticism.

OUTPATIENT RECORDS KEPT BY THE PATIENT

We found the best form of outpatient record to be a single document kept by the patient. Single because if information is dispersed over two or more documents they do not receive equal attention in a rapid consultation. Thus we found that if a child's weight was recorded on a chart on a different piece of paper from that on which clinic notes were recorded (albeit kept in the same plastic envelope) one or the other record sheet was neglected.

Letting the patient keep the record has distinct advantages, because time is saved by not having to hunt for notes when the patient returns to the outpatient department and because information is always available wherever the patient presents, be it at the village, local health centre, or hospital. There is also the advantage of involving patients more directly with their own health: entrusting the record card to the patient implies a degree of respect and trust that can facilitate communication and cooperation with health service staff.

The possible objections to a single document are threefold:

(1) space for writing notes is cramped;

(2) the patient may lose his card;

(3) the patient may read information that it might be better to withhold from him.

For these reasons we experimented with keeping a separate card, which was kept in the hospital, for all those patients who saw a doctor (as opposed to a nurse practitioner). We soon gave this up, however, because it created a sharp distinction between the doctor's and other people's consultations, and on a simple time and motion basis it meant writing notes twice.

On the question of patients losing their cards, our experience is that they are much less likely to do so than most hospital records departments. As for confidentiality, the times when information must be withheld are few. (This last question may be academic with illiterate patients—except that a relative may well read the card).

Thus, with this system, the only patients for whom separate records need to be kept at the hospital are inpatients and those patients who suffer from conditions that need to be brought to the attention of the public health authorities, or whose legal importance requires information to be available in the patient's absence. Examples of these include tuberculosis (because of the need to trace contacts and those who default from treatment);

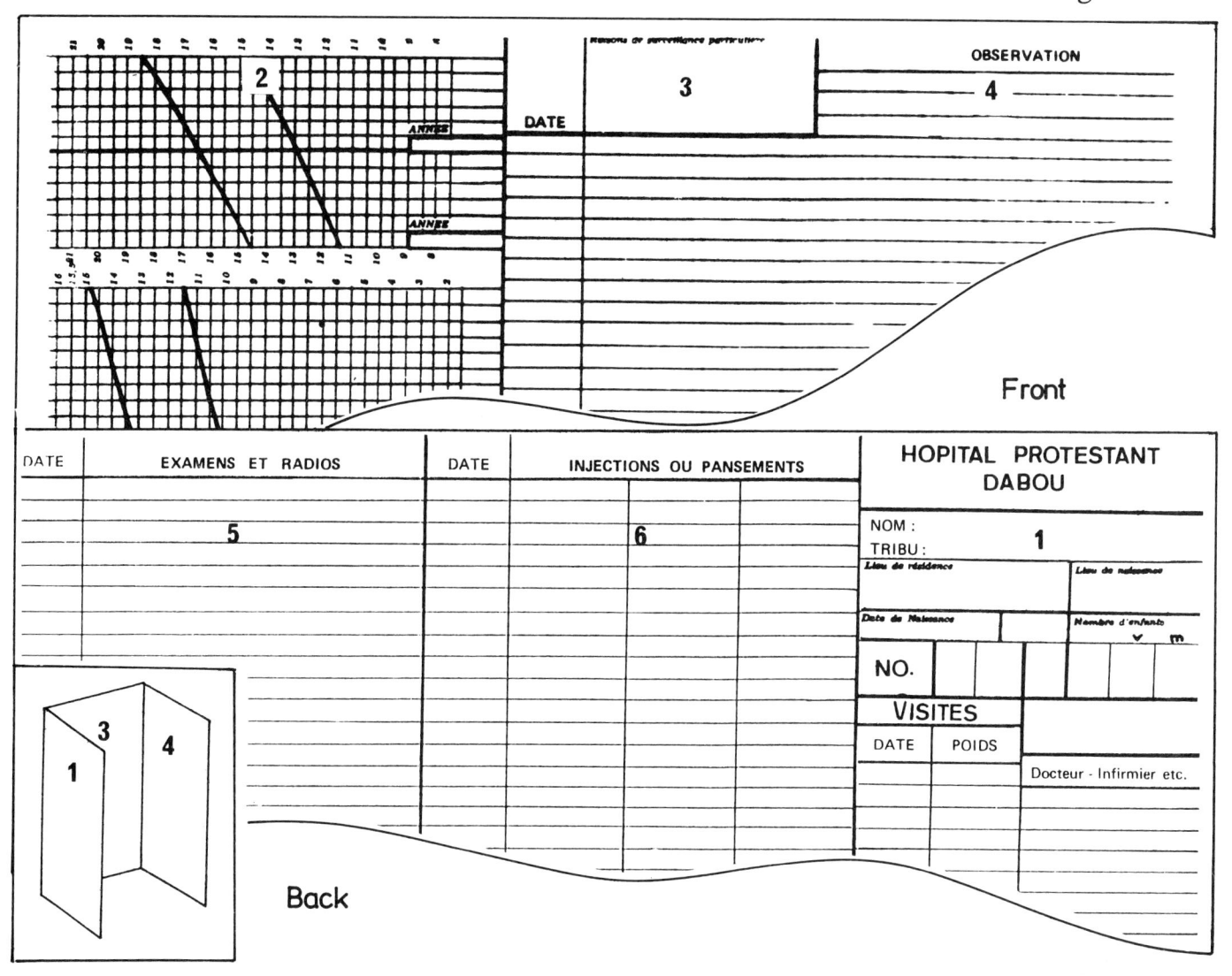

FIG 1—Outpatient record (under 5s version). When folded in three the front becomes sections 2, 3, and 4; the back is sections 5, 6, and 1.

Section 2: Weight chart from birth to 5th birthday; monthly until 3rd birthday, two monthly thereafter. On the four lines at the top, marked by letters A, B, RF, P (B, P, FM, M in English), ticks in the appropriate column indicate that the child is breast feeding, taking maize porridge or an equivalent supplement, sharing in the family meal, and has been given malarial prophylaxis for the coming month.

Section 3 and 4: Clinical notes of each visit. Medicines prescribed and dispensed. At the top of section 3 details of chronic disorders or reasons for the need for special care are recorded.

Section 5: Laboratory tests and requests for x ray films and results.

Section 6: Injections (other than immunisations) and dressings, prescribed and given. Immunisations, set out according to schedule followed locally. Health education given or demonstrations which the mother has attended.

Section 1: Personal details: name, ethnic group, date of birth, places of birth and residence, numbers of living and dead siblings. Clinic attended (hospital, village maternity centre, mobile unit stopping point, etc). Appointments: when, with whom, weight on attendance.

Continuation sheets reproduce and cover sections 3 and 4.

accidents, when prosecution or insurance claims may have to be dealt with; and occupational injury or illness.

The outpatient record cards we devised are shown in figures 1 and 2. They are printed (infants in green, adults in blue) on A4 white card, which is folded in three to make six sections. The card is given to the mother or the patient in a stout protective plastic envelope. When the space available is filled a continuation sheet (duplicated on white paper) is stapled on to form a new notes and prescriptions section. An indefinite number of these sheets may be added, but space must be used economically to avoid ending up with unwieldy bulky records. For routine observations rubber stamps may be used to ensure both completeness and conciseness. The fees (or "frais") section on the adult version, and its absence from the under 5s version, reflects the fact that in the Dabou programme most services for the under 5s are free. Adults pay what they can towards consultations and examinations, and children over 5 pay half price. The weight chart on the under 5s record gives the rough 3rd and 50th centiles (so that mothers can see their child's progress). A good review of the variety of charts used world wide is given by Tremlett et al[2] and is available as a booklet from Teaching Aids at Low Cost.

Patients are told that their record cards are their passport to all the hospital's services and that they need to be shown to every doctor, nurse, or pharmacist consulted. A photograph may be stapled to the adult card to help match cards to patients when these get separated during registration, recording of laboratory examinations, or the dispensing of drugs. We tried to get the patient's registration, consultation, tests, prescribing, and dispensing all completed and recorded within one day. This avoids having to file the record and then retrieve it to record additional information. It also minimises the inconvenience to the patient, who may have had to travel a long distance to reach the hospital.

INPATIENT RECORDS

A single document has advantages for inpatient records, too, for

Writing it down

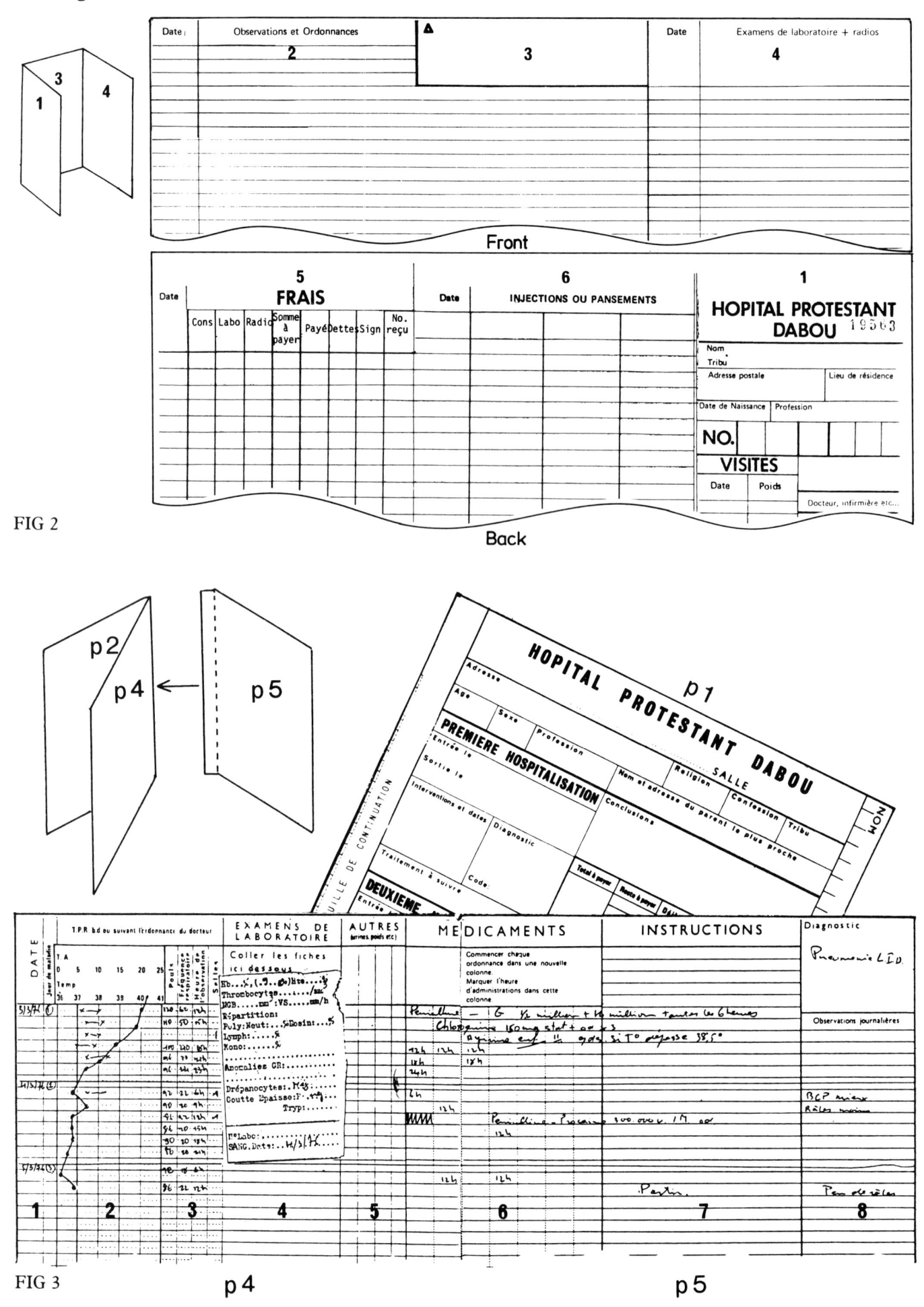

FIG 2

FIG 3

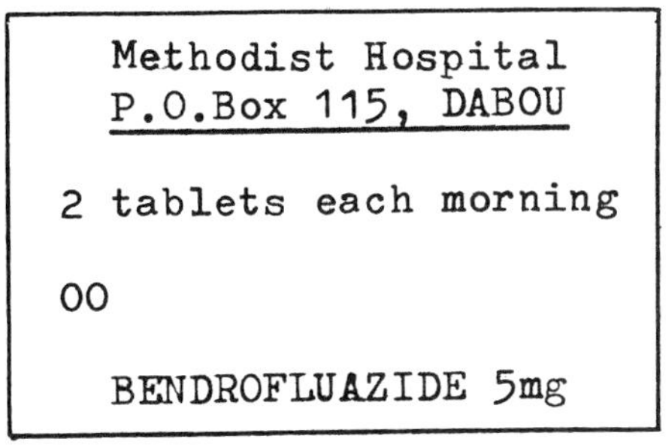

Writing it down

```
┌─────────────────────────────┐
│    Methodist Hospital       │
│    P.O.Box 115, DABOU       │
│                             │
│  2 tablets each morning     │
│                             │
│  oo                         │
│                             │
│     BENDROFLUAZIDE 5mg      │
└─────────────────────────────┘
```

A morning diuretic

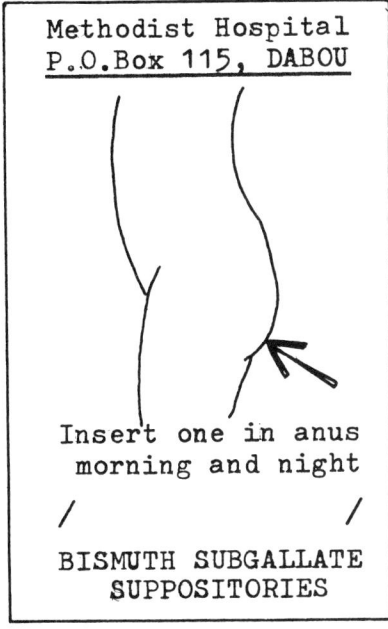

```
┌─────────────────────────────┐
│    Methodist Hospital       │
│    P.O.Box 115, DABOU       │
│                             │
│         (figure)            │
│                             │
│   Insert one in anus        │
│   morning and night         │
│     /         /             │
│                             │
│    BISMUTH SUBGALLATE       │
│       SUPPOSITORIES         │
└─────────────────────────────┘
```

A twice daily suppository

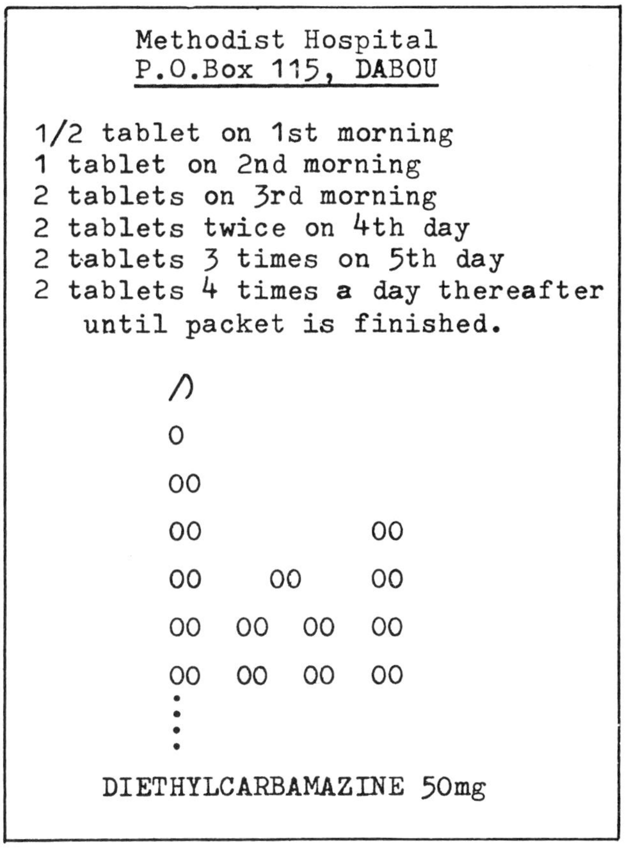

```
┌───────────────────────────────────┐
│      Methodist Hospital           │
│      P.O.Box 115, DABOU           │
│                                   │
│  1/2 tablet on 1st morning        │
│  1 tablet on 2nd morning          │
│  2 tablets on 3rd morning         │
│  2 tablets twice on 4th day       │
│  2 tablets 3 times on 5th day     │
│  2 tablets 4 times a day thereafter│
│     until packet is finished.     │
│                                   │
│              /)                   │
│              o                    │
│              oo                   │
│              oo        oo         │
│              oo   oo   oo         │
│              oo  oo  oo  oo       │
│              oo  oo  oo  oo       │
│                ⋮                  │
│      DIETHYLCARBAMAZINE 50mg      │
└───────────────────────────────────┘
```

A progressive course of diethylcarbamazine

FIG 4—Medicine labels for (a) a morning diuretic, (b) a twice daily suppository, and (c) a progressive course of diethylcarbamazine.

FIG 2 (see facing page)—Outpatient record for adults and children over 5. Front is sections 2, 3, and 4; back sections 5, 6, and 1).
 Sections 2 and 3: Clinical notes at each visit. Medicines prescribed and dispensed. Principal diagnoses are written at top of section 3.
 Section 4: Laboratory tests and requests for x ray films and reports.
 Section 5: Fees charged and paid.
 Section 6: Injections and dressings prescribed and given.
 Section 1: Personal details including blood group and any other information vital in an emergency; appointments: when, with whom, weight on attendance.
 A4 continuation sheets reproduce and cover sections 2, 3, and 4.

FIG 3 (see facing page)—Inpatient record.
 Page 1 (personal details and hospital number). It includes three discharge sections (allowing for three admissions) and boxes for diagnoses, operations, clinical summary, discharge medication, follow up appointments, and payments.
 Page 2 (not illustrated): For use after patient has been discharged. For follow up notes, or for stapling on essential observation charts or details of procedures not included on pages 4 and 5.
 Page 3 (not illustrated): Clinical notes on admission, and any operation notes (recorded in red).
 Pages 4 and 5: Section 1: date, day of hospital stay. Section 2: temperature and blood pressure (different scales on same graph). Section 3: pulse and respiratory rates, time of observation, bowel movements. Section 4: laboratory and x ray examinations. Section 5: four columns for flexible use—for example, regular testing of urine and daily weight. Section 6: prescriptions; each is started on a new line in the first free column, allowing for seven concurrent prescriptions; the nurse writes the time in the appropriate column each time a medicine is given; a prescription is cancelled by hatching a full line under it. Section 7: instructions concerning regimen, diet, intravenous fluids, etc. Section 8: diagnosis, progress notes.
 Page 6: copy of page 4.
 The continuation sheet thus has page 4 on one side and page 5 on the other; adding successive ones reproduces the page 4-5 spread as many times as the length of stay requires; the resulting book is easy to scan and simple to file.

both ease of recording and reading during the patient's stay. It also makes filing and transport simpler once the patient has been discharged home. If the record is to be filed in the hospital it needs to be numbered. The model described below and shown in figure 3 was inspired by that used in Wesley Guild Hospital, Ilesha, Nigeria, and is based on Willis's columnised medical charting.[1] The time axis is vertical, which makes instructions and observations, related to time, easy to follow.

Figure 3 shows that there are six pages; the first four are printed on a single folded A3 card, and the remaining two on a sheet of A4 paper pasted by its margin. The hospital number is based on the date of birth and is compiled from the last two digits of the year of birth and a letter denoting the month of birth (A = January, B = February . . .) for children; for patients first registered as adults this is replaced by Q as the month is unimportant. This is then followed by a three digit serial number. Thus the 37th child to be registered among those born in May 1981 would have the number 81 E 037. Ring binders containing a sheet for each month of birth with the numbers 000-999 on each sheet enable the records clerk to allocate the serial number.

Advice and instructions to patients

The most important communication with any patient is obviously verbal, and it is important to ensure that advice, and instructions on how to take medications, are given to the patients in their own language and idiom. Written instructions are also necessary, however, as a reminder to the patients when they return home,

Writing it down

particularly if several medicines are dispensed. These may be in the national language or in local dialect, but many patients can read neither. We found that the most effective way to get a message across was to combine spoken instructions in dialect with written symbols, whose meaning was first explained to the patients in their own dialect. We experimented, as others have,[3] with labels or notes using a variety of symbols—for example, crowing cocks and setting suns—but in the end found that a simpler system (fig 4) was just as good. This system used the position on the page to indicate the time of day, O to indicate a tablet, D or /\ for half a tablet, and / to indicate a unit of a given treatment. The route of administration (if not oral) was indicated by an accompanying anatomical illustration. This system proved to be cheap because most labels could be typed on a duplicator stencil.

In figure 4 labels for a morning diuretic, a twice daily suppository, and a course of diethylcarbamazine are shown. The last indicates the increasing dose to be taken on successive days, and shows that even complex schedules may be expressed simply. We found that compliance with these instructions was usually good, provided that the meaning of the symbols was carefully explained to the patient.

Labels, such as the ones shown, may be slipped inside transparent sachets. These may be made from rolls of plastic, using a pedal operated heat sealing machine, and allow tablets and even ointments to be dispensed far more cheaply than if commercial packages are used. Moreover, since the sachets or containers contain exactly the number of tablets required, and intelligible instructions, the course is likely to be followed correctly.

A broader study of ways in which suitable containers may be made is planned by the Appropriate Health Resources and Technologies Action Group (AHRTAG).

Standard treatment schedules should be worked out in great detail and copies made available to staff together with step by step aids to diagnosis and management. A book of such schedules, including comparative costs, administrative procedures, and useful contacts, is a godsend to harrassed workers called on to treat patients with unfamiliar diseases: it is a proved antidote to the panic experienced by a physician receiving paediatric or surgical emergencies in the middle of the night. The standardisation of drug regimens also speeds dispensing and allows annual drug needs to be estimated.

An illustrative approach is a good way to convey many other messages—for instance, how to make up and administer oral rehydration fluid. Similarly, dates for immunisations may be suggested by syringes or dropper bottles on the chart and may be filled in by the mother. Colour codes are of limited value because they are expensive to print and some languages recognise only red, white, and black. But colour charts can be invaluable for certain limited purposes, such as helping patients indicate the colour of their sputum or urine, and perhaps linking coded medicines with coded symptoms for illiterate workers.

Like all communication, health education needs thorough testing to avoid misunderstanding. It is salutary to remember the cautionary tale of the villagers who, after an illustrated talk on malarial vector control, remarked how fortunate they were not to be plagued by the giant mosquitoes depicted on the poster.

I am grateful to Dr G J Draper and my Dabou colleagues who developed various stages of the records described; to Dr C A Pearson and Professor D C Morley, who set us on the right road; and to my wife, who, as well as being a colleague, typed the drafts and manuscript of this article.

References

1 Morley D. Medical records. In: King M, ed. *Medical care in developing countries*. Nairobi: Oxford University Press, 1966;**26**:1-12.
2 Tremlett G, Lovel H, Morley D. Guidelines for the design of national weight for age growth charts. *Assignment Children* 1983;**61**:143-75.
3 Ngarama BN, MacDougall JI. To improve a patient's understanding of prescriptions. *Trop Doc* 1975;**5**:135-7.

Useful addresses

Teaching Aids at Low Cost (TALC), PO Box 49, St Albans, Herts AL1 4AX.
Appropriate Health Resources and Technologies Action Group Ltd (AHRTAG), 85 Marylebone High Street, London W1M 3DE.
Samples of Dabou record cards (with full details and an English translation) may be obtained from Dr P H Snell, Hope House, Saltergate Lane, Bamford, Sheffield S30 2BE. (Cost £1.)

INDEX

Amnioscopy 16
Anaesthesia 25–28
   equipment 26
   inhalational 25
   intravenous 27
   intubation 27
   teaching 28
   ventilators 27
Antenatal clinic 15
Appropriateness 1, 8, 35
Asthma 47
Autoclave 3, 32–33

Balance 39
Basic Radiological System (WHO) 9–10
Blair knife 4
Blindness 52–54
   surgery 54
Blood 8
Bronchoscopy 48

Caesarian section 16
Calipers 50
Centrifuge 36
Children. See also Newborn
   mental health 66
   recent developments in care 22
   undernutrition 21
Colorimeter 37, 40, 43
Crosby capsule 41
Crutches 49

Darkroom 10
Delivery, operative 16–17
Disinfection 33
Drugs 55–57
   containers 57
   essential 56
   local manufacture 56

Eclampsia 17
Electrical power 3, 9, 35, 40
Electrocardiograph 43
Emergencies, psychiatric 64
Endoscopy 41, 48

Fetal monitors 16
Flame photometer 40
Fluid replacement 7

Growth charts 22

Haemoglobin meter 37
Haemorrhage 17
Health education 58–60
Heat block 25
Hepatitis B vaccine 41

Immunisation 6–7, 23
Incubator 39
Infections 46–47
Intensive care, neonatal 20
Intubation 27

Kidney dishes 4

Laboratory equipment 35–39
Labour ward 16
Low birth weight 18

Maintenance 12–14
   preventive 13
   staff 12
Measles immunisation 6
Mental health 64–67
Microscope 36, 40, 43

Neuroses 65
Newborn
   care of 18–20
   infections 18
   intensive care 20
   low birth weight 18
   problems in first week 20
   resuscitation 19
Newsletters 61
Nutrition 21, 22
   parenteral 41
   undernutrition in children 21

Operating theatre 3–5
   instruments 4
   lighting 3
   table 4
Oral rehydration 7–8, 22

PATH (Program for Appropriate Technology in health) 8
Patients
   advice to 71
   records 68
Pattern of disease 29

Pleural disease 48
Population estimation 30
Preventive services 21

Record keeping 68–72
Research 29–31
Refrigeration 6
   solar powered 1
Refrigerator 38, 40
Respiratory infections 46
Resuscitation of neonate 17, 19

Sandals 49
Sewage disposal 32
Silver swaddler 1
Solar powered refrigeration 1
Spectacles 54
Sterilisation 32–33
Steriliser 38
Sterility 3
Stethoscope 43
Stills 8
Surgery
   allocating funds 3
   cardiac 45
   ophthalmic 54
Symphysiotomy 16

Tally survey 28
Teaching aids 61–63
Tetanus 16, 18

Ultrasound 11
Undernutrition 21

Vaccine safety marker 1
Ventilators 27

Waste disposal 32
Water bath 37
Water still 38
Water supply 32
World Health Organisation Basic Radiological System 9

X rays
   equipment 9–11, 43
   films and cassettes 10